Pain-Related Fear

Mission Statement of IASP Press®

The International Association for the Study of Pain (IASP) brings together scientists, clinicians, health care providers, and policy makers to stimulate and support the study of pain and to translate that knowledge into improved pain relief worldwide. IASP Press publishes timely, high-quality, and reasonably priced books relating to pain research and treatment.

Pain-Related Fear
Exposure-Based Treatment
for Chronic Pain

Johan W.S. Vlaeyen, PhD
Research Group Health Psychology, Faculty of Psychology and Educational Sciences, University of Leuven, Belgium; Department of Clinical Psychological Science, Faculty of Psychology and Neuroscience, Maastricht University, The Netherlands

Stephen J. Morley, MPhil, PhD
Institute of Health Sciences, University of Leeds, and Department of Clinical Health Psychology, St James' University Hospital, Leeds, United Kingdom

Steven J. Linton, PhD
Center for Health and Medical Psychology, Örebrö University, Örebrö, Sweden

Katja Boersma, PhD
Center for Health and Medical Psychology, Örebrö University, Örebrö, Sweden

Jeroen de Jong, PhD
Department of Rehabilitation, Maastricht University Hospital, Maastricht, The Netherlands

IASP PRESS® ♦ SEATTLE

First printing, 2012
Cover design by Lori Wardian

Library of Congress Cataloging-in-Publication Data

Library of Congress Control Number: 2012028388

Published by:
IASP Press®
International Association for the Study of Pain
111 Queen Anne Ave N, Suite 501
Seattle, WA 98109-4955, USA
Fax: 206-283-9403
www.iasp-pain.org

Printed in the United States of America

Contents

Contents of Book

Contents of DVD

Therapist Materials
1. Understanding Behavioral Experiments
2. Behavioral Experiment Form
3. Guidelines for Behavioral Experiments
4. Complicating Factors of In Vivo Exposure Treatment

Patient Materials
5. General Information
6. The Vicious Cycle
7. Patient Information About Treatment
8. Understanding Behavioral Experiments
9. Strategies for Preventing a Relapse

Videos
1. Intake
2. Education Session
3. Establishing a Fear Hierarchy
4. Exposure in Behavioral Experiments: Climbing Stairs
5. Exposure in Behavioral Experiments: Lifting
6. Exposure in Behavioral Experiments: Bicycling
7. Evaluation of the Exposure Treatment

Preface

The idea for this book began with a conversation between two of us (Johan Vlaeyen and Stephen Morley) about how to disseminate the treatment based on the fear-avoidance model that had been developed in Maastricht (the Netherlands) by Johan Vlaeyen, Jeroen de Jong, and their colleagues, and further tested by the Örebro group (Steven Linton, Katja Boersma, and their colleagues) in Sweden. The Maastricht group had developed a manual for use in a randomized controlled trial [1], but it was only available in Dutch [2], and Morley asked whether an English version was available. Our initial thought was simply to prepare a translation of this manual, but we were aware that many clinicians who might be interested in the treatment might also value a more extended introduction to the theoretical basis of the treatment. When we discussed the idea further, we added a wish list that included providing users with guidance on how to evaluate their own implementation and some resources to use. Hence, the idea for this book was born.

We are grateful to IASP for taking on the project, and we thank the the IASP publications staff for their great patience and understanding, especially Elizabeth Endres and Kathy Havers and latterly Ivar Nelson in the IASP office, and Cathy Bushnell and Maria Adele Giamberardino as the IASP officers.

The project has had a longer gestation than we initially planned because we "slightly" overestimated the demands placed on each of us. Morley drafted chapters 1, 6, 7, and 8, and Vlaeyen drafted chapters 2, 3, and 4. Boersma drafted chapter 5 and SL chapter 9. Each chapter was commented on and contributed to by all authors. de Jong's invaluable hands-on clinical expertise not only enabled him to make major contributions to the text but can also be seen on the accompanying DVD. His immense clinical skill makes treatment look unbelievably simple. We ask readers not to be deceived by appearances. If you do decide to introduce the methods reported in this text, we strongly advise that you work as a team and receive supervision from a qualified cognitive-behavioral therapist who has experience of behavioral exposure in clinical settings.

It is not surprising that learning theory models of fear and avoidance have dominated the field of psychopathology in relation to phobias,

[1] Leeuw M, Goossens ME, van Breukelen GJ, de Jong JR, Heuts PH, Smeets RJ, Koke AJ, Vlaeyen JW. Exposure in vivo versus operant graded activity in chronic low back pain patients: results of a randomized controlled trial. Pain 2008;138:192–207.

[2] Leeuw M, Vlaeyen JWS, de Jong JR, Goossens MEJB. Behandelprotocol exposure in vivo bij chronische lage rugpijn. Amsterdam: Boom; 2006.

anxiety, obsessive-compulsive behavior, and related problems. But until recently, fear-avoidance has been far from mainstream thinking about how to provide treatment for chronic pain patients. When Vlaeyen and Morley were discussing the book project, we noted that each of us had been influenced by a significant figure in this field. Vlaeyen had spent a year with the late Bill Fordyce in Washington in the 1980s and had been profoundly influenced by his powerful concepts and ideas. Fordyce was not only a superb mentor, but taught us—among many insights—the crucial difference between "hurt" and "harm" with respect to chronic pain. Often patients who experience pain avoid physical activity as they are convinced that the pain associated with movement signals the presence of bodily damage. Although not recognized by many, one of the strengths of Bill Fordyce's clinical approach was his ability to use metaphors in his educational session with patients to elucidate the mechanisms of learning. For example, Bill talked about the painful movement of the arm after successful healing of a bone fracture to illustrate that pain can be a result of muscle weakness (immobility due to the cast) rather than injury. We decided to extend Fordyce's work in identifying such fear of movement and injury as a primary issue in chronic pain management, and design a treatment systematically targeting these fears. Morley completed his PhD studies under the guidance and tutelage of Clare Philips, who had begun to apply ideas of fear-avoidance initially in the field of headache and then more generally. Her kindly influence has for many years remained a model of how to stimulate and supervise students.

Our respect for both Bill and Clare is immense, and as an expression of deep appreciation we would like to dedicate this book to the memory of the late Bill Fordyce and to Clare Philips. Thank you, both of you.

We would also like to thank all of our colleagues and members of the interdisciplinary treatment teams we have successfully worked with over the past few years. We are grateful for the fruitful collaborations and numerous and inspiring discussions. We also thank our patients with chronic pain for their confidence and for their help in developing the exposure in vivo treatment, even they may not have been aware of their contribution. Vlaeyen was supported by the Odysseus Grant "The Psychology of Pain and Disability Research Program" funded by the Research Foundation, Flanders, Belgium (FWO Vlaanderen), and by the University of Leuven Center of Excellence on Generalization Research in Ill Health and Psychopathology (GRIPP).

Johan W.S. Vlaeyen, Stephen Morley, Steven J. Linton, Katja Boersma, and Jeroen de Jong
March 2012, Leuven, Leeds, Örebro, and Maastricht

The Context of the Fear-Avoidance Model

The aim of this chapter is to provide an introduction to the fear-avoidance model as applied to a particular problem in the psychology of pain—the relationship between movement-related pain and the fearful anticipation of its consequences. We will explore the model in some detail in subsequent chapters, but the aim of this chapter is to establish the context in which the fear-avoidance model was developed. The fear-avoidance model is a recent application of important psychological principles that have been used to solve a variety of problems relating to fear over the past 50 to 60 years. Although research into the fear-avoidance model of pain has grown considerably in the past few years, it is a relatively recent arrival on the main stage of our efforts to apply psychological principles to the relief of pain and its unwanted consequences.

In the first part of this chapter, we briefly review the development of contemporary psychological treatments of chronic pain. This review has two purposes. First, it contextualizes the fear-avoidance model. In doing so, we aim to draw out the distinctive features of this approach to the treatment of pain. Second, we note that the principles of the fear-avoidance model have been applied to one particular problem in chronic pain, but it is possible to apply the general model to other aspects of pain experience and behavior. We will explore some of these aspects in the final chapter. Of course, modern attempts to apply psychological principles to mental health problems have historical roots [16], and contemporary approaches to problems of excessive fear and anxiety draw extensively on the application of learning theory [17]. Therefore, in the second part of the chapter, we briefly review the application of learning theory to problems of anxiety in the general area of mental health and highlight lessons learned and advances in the field overall.

Contemporary Psychological Treatments of Pain

Cognitive-behavioral therapy (CBT) is the dominant force in contemporary psychological treatments for chronic pain [34]. We will explore a general definition of CBT a little later in this chapter, but we note here that Gatchel and colleagues [21] provide a discussion of CBT with regard to the field of chronic pain. They note that, "CBT techniques proceed from the view that an individual's interpretation, evaluation, and beliefs about his or her health condition and coping repertoire, with respect to pain and disability, will affect the degree of emotional and physical disability associated with the pain condition." In addition, "It should also be noted that the usage of the term *cognitive behavioral therapy* varies widely and may include self-instructions (e.g., distraction, imagery, motivational self-talk), relaxation or biofeedback, development of coping strategies (e.g., increasing assertiveness, minimizing of negative self-defeating thoughts), changing dysfunctional beliefs about pain, and goal setting. A patient referred for CBT may be exposed to varying selections of these strategies. Finally, it should also be pointed out that these CBT techniques are embedded in more comprehensive pain management programs that also include functional restoration, pharmacotherapy, and general medical management." The salient feature of this commentary is the attempt to capture the broad definition of CBT as applied to chronic pain in two ways. First, Gatchel and colleagues provide only the most general statement regarding the central component of cognitive appraisal, so that there is no specific, precise model that would allow a working clinician to map a patient's experience onto specific therapeutic procedures linked to particular outcomes. Second, they list a wide range of therapeutic activities and note that these appear in varying mixtures in different research and clinical protocols. Gatchel and colleagues are not alone in noting the broad definition of CBT and its relative lack of specificity [for example, see references 13, 35, and 53]. This definition does capture the breadth of CBT, the mixture of techniques, aims, and the variation in the context in which CBT is practiced. To understand some of the key elements, it is useful to see how the main strands have developed, and where they have been incorporated into the field of pain.

Table I shows a timeline that broadly schematizes the major strands of contemporary CBT for chronic pain. The major schools that have contributed are shown in bold typeface, and their theoretical or practical antecedents are shown in italic typeface. We locate the beginning of contemporary psychological treatment with the application of behavior analysis by Fordyce and colleagues in the 1960s [19,20] and ending with the introduction of acceptance and commitment therapy (ACT) in the late 1990s and from 2000 onward [32]. Both Fordyce's application of operant principles and ACT have their roots in Skinner's work on behavior analysis (also termed operant behavior analysis) originating in the 1930s [45]. Behavior analysis seeks to understand the laws that determine how an individual learns the relationship between two events, that is, their own behavior and its consequences. Behavior analysis considers that behavior is a function of two significant classes of predominantly external factors. The first class, reinforcement, refers to consequences that determine the future probability of a specific behavior. There are four fundamental types of reinforcement; two increase the probability of the preceding behavior (positive and negative reinforcers), and two decrease the probability of the preceding behavior (punishment and extinction). The second class, antecedents, refers to the context in which behavior occurs and includes the presence of discriminative stimuli (S^D) that signal the availability of reinforcement. The influences of the two principles in governing behavior have been investigated extensively for more than 70 years in both laboratory and real-world settings and offer powerful methods for influencing behavior [42]. Fordyce's insight was to recognize that although pain is essentially a private experience, there are publicly observable expressions of pain that are subject to the influences of reinforcement and the context in which it occurs. As a consequence, behavior occurring with the presence of pain may be modified in many ways, of which some are unhelpful. Fordyce argued that it is possible to use the technical knowledge

Table I
Timeline outlining the development of cognitive-behavioral therapy as applied to the treatment of chronic pain

1940	1960	1970	1980	1990	2000
Operant behavior analysis	**Operant therapy**	**Biofeedback**	**Cognitive therapy**	**Fear-avoidance model**	**Acceptance and commitment therapy**
	Pavlovian conditioning	**Stress management**	**Mindfulness-based stress reduction**	*Behavior analysis of language*	
	1. Cognitive theory of stress				
	2. Behavioral analysis of self-control				
	Clinical observations				
Mowrer-Miller two-process theory					
Buddhism (1000 BCE)					

Source: Adapted from Morley [34].
Note: Major schools are shown in boldface, and their antecedents are shown in italics.

of reinforcement schedules and discriminative stimuli to analyze pain be-havior, and using the same principles of reinforcement and modifying the stimulus control, the behavior can be changed. In a series of elegant exper-imental studies in human subjects, Fordyce and colleagues demonstrated the therapeutic possibilities of reinforcement and stimulus control. One result of this was the demonstration of the importance of reinforcement and stimulus control arising from an individual's social environment. As a result, many pain management protocols include sessions focused on modifying family interactions with an operant protocol.

Acceptance and commitment therapy emerged in the 1990s as a practical consequence of a radical behavioral analysis of the function of lan-guage and rule-governed behavior [13,22,32]. This account recognizes that the relationship between behavior and its consequences can be captured as rule-governed behavior and expressed in language. Moreover, language has the power to form relations in arbitrary ways that are not necessarily reflected in reality. The central feature of ACT analysis is that an individ-ual's language history can lead them to a state of "psychological inflexibil-ity" such that they are unable to engage in meaningful valued activity and are dominated by their pain experience. They respond to the presence of pain rather than to other contingencies that would allow them to engage in more valued and fulfilling activities. The aim of ACT is to facilitate the individual's engagement with a range of valued activities in the presence of pain. The complexity of ACT is more difficult to grasp than Fordyce's earlier implementation, but in essence the aims are essentially the same; to change the control over behavior that pain exerts by altering the context. It is also important to note that both Fordyce's implementation of operant principles and ACT eschew the control of pain as a focus of treatment. Both treatments deliberately attend to other aspects of the condition of chronic pain. This is a salient feature of most psychological approaches to pain. They do not attempt to deliver analgesia by psychological means but to facilitate a more functional set of responses to the presence of chronic pain that are compatible with reduced distress. Having stated that analgesia is not an aim of psychological treatment, there are psychological approach-es that have, at least in initial instances, focused on pain reduction. In addi-tion, a number of psychological treatments have resulted in pain reduction, even though they were not primarily aimed at analgesia.

By the beginning of the 1970s, biofeedback and relaxation had been introduced into treatment protocols. Biofeedback also had its roots in the analysis of learning. Basic experimental studies were concerned with a particular distinction between classical, or Pavlovian, conditioning (that is, the learning of relationships between stimuli) and (operant) conditioning (that is, the learning of relationships betweenstimuli ans preceding behavior). It was hypothesized that autonomic responses that were normally the focus of Pavlovian conditioning could not be operantly conditioned [33]. Paradoxically, the first applications of biofeedback for pain disorder appear to have been for chronic tension headache and were targeted to striated muscle [9], normally thought to be under volitional control. However, both biofeedback and progressive muscle relaxation were incorporated into treatments for pain. A *pain-tension-pain* cycle was hypothesized as a major process facilitating the maintenance of pain. It was suggested that biofeedback and relaxation could specifically interrupt this cycle, in addition to any nonspecific effects that the treatments might have on the individual's general well-being.

The recognition that chronic pain might be considered a stressor in its own right and that many features of an individual's response can be construed as instrumental and ineffective components of a stress response were also developed in the 1970s. Elements of this analysis were drawn from work in the preceding decade that sought to elucidate factors responsible for the variation in responses to aversive stimuli (stressors) by Lazarus and Folkman [28]. This work established two crucial ideas in the field of pain, appraisal and coping, which are still current (e.g., catastrophizing and coping skills training). In essence, many of the behaviors associated with chronic pain were viewed as ineffective coping strategies that led the individual to a state of hopelessness and despair. Also by the mid-1970s, work on self-control, with roots in behavior analysis [30], was incorporated into the treatment armamentarium, and a definitive text, *Pain and Behavioral Medicine: A Cognitive-Behavioral Perspective*, was published in 1983 [47]. Keefe and colleagues developed a robust pain coping skills protocol [27] as a generic treatment protocol that has been successfully applied to several diagnostic groups. This protocol is entirely coherent with the "pain as stress" model. The major aim of the program is to help patients "reconceptualise their pain and their own ability to control pain" ([27] p. 240). The coping skills training (CST) program includes an initial educational component based around the insight of Melzack and Wall's gate control theory, in which the experience of pain is complexly determined and includes top-down influences that can both exacerbate and ameliorate the experience of pain. This generates the rationale for developing strategies that change the individual's primary and secondary appraisals of their pain experience. The roles of persistent rehearsal and practice of adaptive behavior and cognitive strategies is emphasized, and specific coping skills are taught. These include relaxation, rest-activity cycling—which teaches patients to manage their behavioral activity in a time-contingent rather than a pain-contingent manner—and pragmatic attention-diversion strategies to help patients manage situations in which pain increases. The protocol also pays careful attention to preparing patients for life after treatment, with sessions on skills necessary for maintenance. More recently Keefe and colleagues have established the value of posttreatment computerized maintenance sessions delivered by telephone [37].

Toward the end of the 1970s, A.T. Beck and colleagues published an enormously influential text on the treatment of depression by cognitive therapy [4]. The significance of this was that a substantive claim was made that a disorder that had previously been difficult to treat by psychological methods was tractable with clinical techniques that focused on the patient's idiosyncratic thinking about their relationships to current events. Aaron Beck and Albert Ellis had developed separate versions of what became known as cognitive therapy over the previous two decades. The treatment was grounded in acute clinical observation rather than fundamental laboratory experimentation, coupled with a willingness to devise and test treatment tactics in a clinical setting. Experimental analyses of elements of cognitive therapy emerged in conjunction with later randomized controlled trials of Beck's therapy. Perhaps because of the marked overlap between pain and depression elements of Beck's therapy, these elements were incorporated into pain treatments, and the model was adapted to the treatment of chronic pain [46]. Cognitive therapy emphasized the critical mediational role played by idiosyncratic interpretations of events in determining an individual's emotional and behavioral responses to an event. The model included a structural analysis of dysfunctional thinking and hypothesized a developing underlying schema and modes of information processing. There is no doubt that that Beck's 20-session protocol for treating depression is effective [10]. Interestingly, subsequent analyses have indicated that improvements in depression often begin before the introduction of the major cognitive components of treatment and occur in the first stages, when patients are engaged in a behavioral activation program [14,24,31]. The roots of behavioral activation lie in an earlier behavioral analysis of depression [18] that emphasizes lack of reinforcement and the prevalence of *passive* avoidance strategies, that is, *not* doing something to avoid unwanted consequences. There is good evidence that in their own right, behavioral activation programs are effective for treating depression [14,15,50].

Central to the clinical implementation of cognitive therapy are the ideas of automatic thoughts and core beliefs. The link between these ideas and the stress coping model is apparent, and in the literature it is not always possible to separate the "pure" implementations of each type of treatment and comprehensive pain management programs might well include elements from both models. Thorn [46] provides an example of a cognitive therapy approach to chronic pain that, while avowedly influenced by Beck's model and therapeutic approach, is also embedded within the stress-appraisal model. The program begins by helping patients establish the relationship between personal stressors and exacerbation of their pain experience. Central to this is the focus on the patient's appraisal of the stressful event in terms of the challenges, threats, and losses that the event implies. The central cognitive component of automatic thoughts is invoked as the crucial link between the event and the individual's response to it. Patients are taught to notice and capture the fleeting images and thoughts that occur in the context of a stressor. For example, an increase in pain (a stressor in its own right) might be accompanied by an image of themselves writhing in agony and the fleeting thought, "This pain will get worse and never end." Careful exploration of the thoughts and images can be used to illustrate their influence on the experience of pain (generally incremental), and patients are taught to evaluate the consequences and test the veracity of their thoughts with a structured self-monitoring protocol and by developing alternative evaluations that can be tested via small, targeted behavioral experiments. The aim of these interventions is to change the patient's evaluation of their habitual responses to pain and to change the behavioral consequences of these appraisals. The second strand of cognitive therapy is to identify general beliefs (also called "core beliefs" or "cognitive schemas") that are hypothesized to underlie the automatic thoughts and reactions to pain. These beliefs are identified by further exploration and analysis of the automatic thoughts. Statements that include imperatives such as "must," "should," or "ought" often characterize the beliefs. As with negative automatic thoughts, the evidential basis and functional consequences for each belief are explored, and patients are guided toward developing alternative, more functional beliefs that can be subjected to further evaluation. Given the significant association between depression and chronic pain, it should not be surprising that Beck's approach to cognitive therapy was incorporated into pain management protocols. Although there are specific focused cognitive therapy protocols, such as Thorn's [46], examination of the description of many published accounts of CBT for pain suggests that what has been introduced into treatment is a range of ideas and techniques from mainstream cognitive therapy, perhaps in a somewhat limited manner. This makes the evaluation "pure" cognitive therapy for chronic pain somewhat problematic.

A second strand of treatment, mindfulness, also without roots in experimental psychology, was also introduced in the mid-1980s. Kabat-Zinn [25] reported uncontrolled evaluations of the application of mindfulness training derived from 3000 years of Buddhist teaching and practice. Although Kabat-Zinn reported studies on patients with pain, it was not until his work was taken up by a group of researchers looking for a method to prevent relapse after treatment for depression [53] that mindfulness was incorporated more generally into CBT. Evaluations of mindfulness training for chronic pain, both generally and as exemplified in specific conditions, are now being published [36,55], as are laboratory studies of its effects. Although there are several definitions of mindfulness discussed in the literature, key aspects are a present-moment, nonreactive, and non-judgmental awareness, thereby disengaging from (the need for) control and specific (achievement) goals [8]. Importantly, mindful awareness is flexible, self-regulated, and does not involve conceptual processing [6]. In a mindful state, pain sensations are considered for only what they are, without giving them a particular meaning. For example, Schutze and colleagues [43] demonstrated that mindfulness uniquely predicts more pain

catastrophizing and also moderates the relationship between pain intensity and pain catastrophizing. Outpatients with chronic pain who scored
low on a standardized measure of mindfulness (compared to those who
scored high) reported more catastrophic interpretations of pain when experiencing high pain levels.

The Psychological Treatment of Fears and Phobias: A Brief Overview

Before we consider the fear-avoidance model of pain in detail, we will take
a small detour to consider the background for the development of this
model. Attempts to understand fear and its clinical manifestations, phobias, have a long and intricate history in the field of psychology and psychiatry. The majority of contemporary treatments are derived from attempts
to understand factors relating to the genesis and maintenance of fear and
thus shape how interventions may target these factors for therapeutic benefit [41]. At the start of the 20th century, the psychoanalytic account that
was to dominate treatment for the next 50 to 60 years emerged. This subtle
and complex account conceptualized pathological states of fear as arising
from disturbed normal psychological development rooted in intrapsychic
conflict. At its essence was the notion that particular phobias were symbolic representations of this conflict and that their function was to shield
the individual from the psychological pain inherent in the conflict. Treatment was a long and costly process in which the symbolic meaning of
the phobia was uncovered and the conflict resolved [16]. Yet, at the same
time that this clinically based theory and treatment was being developed
and implemented, Pavlov was conducting laboratory experiments exploring the development of fear and neurotic-like behavior in animals using
his conditioning paradigm, and Watson and Rayner [51] published a fa-
mous study applying Pavlovian conditioning to establish fear of a white
rat in a young boy who had not previously shown any fear of the rat (it
is doubtful that this experiment would be ethically sanctioned today).
The clinical implications and consequences of this work and further experimental studies carried out in the 1930s and 1940s by, among others,
Mowrer and Miller, did not fully emerge until 1958 with the publication
of *Psychotherapy by Reciprocal Inhibition* by Joseph Wolpe [54]. Wolpe

reported on an extensive case series of patients with a range of phobias, which he had successfully treated with a new method called "systematic desensitization."

Joseph Wolpe, a South African psychiatrist, regarded his experience of treating psychologically traumatized soldiers in World War II as unsatisfactory [40]. On return to civilian life, he began to consider ways in which he might establish a model of fear and avoidance. In the laboratory, he established fear and avoidance behavior in cats with the use of a simple Pavlovian task in which the animals received an electric shock if they approached a specific location in the experimental room. By this means, the cats acquired spatial avoidance and fear, that is, they avoided this location and showed typical feline displays of fear if placed in this location. Wolpe now had a model of phobia; the next step was to develop a formal treatment to reverse the fear and avoidance. In the laboratory, Wolpe's treatment had two essential elements; first, *graded* and *gradual* exposure to the feared location. The treatment was graded because Wolpe used decreasing spatial proximity to the feared location, and it was gradual because a change in proximity was only made when the animal showed no sign of anxiety at the current test location. The animals only moved up the fear hierarchy once signs of fear had decreased. The second element was to inhibit expression of fear by simultaneously presenting a stimulus that would generate a motivational state incompatible with fear—termed reciprocal inhibition. Wolpe found that by using this strategy, it was possible to train animals to visit the feared location without displaying fear.

In translating this protocol for the clinic, Wolpe had to solve two significant problems. First, many human fears cannot be represented by a simple spatial location, and there are many subtle changes in stimulus conditions with variations in fear. In addition, it was impossible to recreate this variation in the clinic, given that it would have required Wolpe to have an extensive set of theatrical props to recreate the range of feared environments. The second problem was to determine a suitable stimulus to act as a reciprocal inhibitor of fear. Unfettered access to food, alcohol, and other motivational stimuli had obvious disadvantages. The solution to these problems was to present the feared stimulus by carefully describing it and asking the patient to construct an image and to train the patient in progressive muscle relaxation. The treatment therefore involved presenting a representation of the feared stimulus while the patient was in a state of relaxation. The images were visualized for relatively short periods of time (5–10 seconds), slowly ascending the fear hierarchy so that the patient did not experience fear in the presence of the stimulus.

Wolpe's reported high success rate for this treatment (90%) was impressive and his protocol explicit and reproducible. Furthermore, he proposed, at least on the face of it, a testable theoretical account of the change process. Within a relatively short period of time, systematic desensitization was subjected to considerable clinical and experimental scrutiny, giving rise to some of the first randomized clinical trials of a psychological treatment. The fact that the protocol was apparently simple and that the model was applicable to fear in general, rather than to specific psychopathological states, meant that is was possible to conduct laboratory studies on a wide range of common "normal" fears found in the population. One consequence of adopting the behavioral learning theory approach was that clinical manifestations of fear were regarded as essentially the product of normal psychological processes related to Pavlovian and operant conditioning rather than the consequence of a pathological interruption of psychological development.

Laboratory studies tested the tenets of systematic desensitization, extensively asking several key questions. For example, is it necessary to present the feared stimulus in a hierarchy? Does one need an explicit counter-conditioning state? Is longer actual presentation of the feared object as effective as shorter imagined presentation? The answer to many of these questions was generally, "No" [26,39]. Although there were clinical circumstances in which graded, gradual exposure in the context of explicit relaxation were advantageous, for example when needing to motivate highly fearful patients to engage their fears, it was also clear that direct and sometimes prolonged exposure to the actual feared event (in vivo exposure) without a hierarchy or relaxation could be therapeutically effective [7]. Indeed, direct, in vivo exposure became the preferred option for most behavioral treatment protocols for fear and anxiety, and it is only recently that the role of imagery in maintaining and treating anxiety states has been reappraised and subjected to experimental scrutiny [23].

Although Wolpe's systematic desensitization relied overtly on cognitive processes, for example the patient's report to establish the fear hierarchy and the use of images in treatment, there was no overt attempt to directly change the cognitive element of the treatment or to consider an explanation of the effectiveness of the treatment according to cognitive constructs. With respect to the latter, change in fearfulness was deemed to occur in a relatively automatic, nonconscious way by the process of reciprocal inhibition. At the theoretical level, reciprocal inhibition turned out to be a slippery construct, and an alternative model based on the physiology of habituation, "maximal habituation," was proposed. It too proved to be difficult to test because there was no independent measure of habituation other than the decrease in anxiety response–the very thing it set out to explain [52]. We will return to the theory behind fear reduction at a later point.

As we noted earlier, the basis of what was to become cognitive therapy emerged in the 1960s and 1970s, marked by the publication of Beck's monograph on depression [4]. Beck had also worked with fear and anxiety, and his analysis of his clinical observations clearly articulated a key component of cognitive therapy, which was that every disorder was characterized by a specific pattern of cognitive appraisal [3]. Arguably, it was the development of a cognitive model of panic disorder that essentially captured the essence of both a cognitive account of a disorder and clinical and therapeutic implications. Very similar accounts were proposed by David Clark [11] in the United Kingdom and David H. Barlow [2] in the United States. Clark's cognitive analysis is shown diagrammatically in Fig. 1.

Clark proposed that patients with repeated panic attacks have a predisposition to interpret certain bodily sensations in a catastrophic fashion. The sensations, such as breathlessness, palpitations, and dizziness, are those associated with *normal* apprehension and anxiety. Rather than accept the sensations for what they are, the individual with panic interprets them as indicative of great danger and impending disaster, thus further fueling anxiety. For example, the following interpretations of the symptoms of breathlessness, shaking, and palpitations are possible:

Breathlessness means: "My breathing will stop and I will die."
Shaking means: "I am losing control and will become insane."
Palpitations mean: "A heart attack is impending and I will die."

Clark proposed that some event initially acts as a trigger to elicit symptoms giving rise to a feeling of apprehension. At least one of the symptoms is then interpreted catastrophically and elevates the perceived threat. This elevation may be followed by further symptoms and further catastrophic interpretations as the process enters into a vicious cycle that perpetuates the attack. Clark argued that the model could be applied to explain both attacks preceded by a sense of heightened anxiety, common for example in agoraphobic patients leaving a place of presumed safety, and attacks that came "out of the blue." All that the model requires is that the patient experiences a meaningful bodily sensation that can then be interpreted as catastrophic. Any event that increases the probability of such an event (heightened emotions, excessive caffeine intake, hyperventilation, hemodynamic postural adjustments leading to dizziness) may give rise to the experience.

The initial model led to four testable propositions as follows: (1) patients with panic attacks are more likely to (mis)interpret bodily sensations in a catastrophic fashion, (2) activating catastrophic (mis)interpretations will induce a panic attack, (3) panic attacks may be reduced by decreasing catastrophic interpretations, and (4) sustained therapeutic

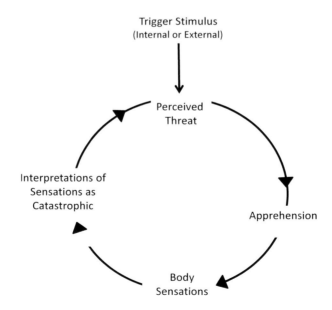

Fig. 1. A simple schematic representation of Clark's cognitive-behavioral model for panic disorder (see text for explanation).

improvements (whatever the treatment) will be determined by the extent to which catastrophic (mis)interpretations are changed. Clark provided evidence for each of these propositions, and subsequent research has generally supported the model [1].

For our purposes, there are several essential features of Clark's cognitive formulation that have a bearing on the fear-avoidance model of pain. First is the realization that although many anxiety disorders have catastrophic thinking associated with them (i.e., it is a common process), the content of the appraisal will contain a theme specific to the disorder that will shape the subsequent avoidance pattern. For example, social anxiety is dominated by appraisal of others making negative evaluations of one's actions or presentation [12]. The relationship between specific appraisals and the behavioral phenotypes of different anxiety states has been a fruitful field of clinical research, and many specific models have emerged. In this regard, the fear-avoidance model of pain is one such model.

The second feature of the cognitive model of panic, and hence of most cognitive models, is a subtle departure from the earlier behavioral model vis-à-vis the way in which treatment is planned and delivered. The behavioral model requires that the therapist develop a hierarchy on the basis of a gradient of fear. Subsequent exposure to the hierarchy results in a relatively automatic weakening of the power of specific situations to elicit the fear response. The skill of the therapist is therefore in determining the gradual incremental nature of the hierarchy and in ensuring that it captures all of the relevant stimulus components that contribute to the elicitation of fear. In contrast, Clark's model of panic requires the therapist to identify specific thoughts and appraisals associated with events and situations that elicit the fear response. Because these thoughts and appraisals are hypothesized to have a functional relationship with subsequent behavior, it follows that the third distinguishing feature is that treatment is directed toward challenging the veracity of the patient's beliefs and predictions by giving them structured opportunities to reappraise these beliefs and predictions. The focus of treatment is therefore to devise individualized behavioral experiments that allow the patient to test their beliefs [5]. Needless to say, behavioral experiments frequently include an element of graded exposure, but this is not necessarily so. Verbal challenge of a belief, along with education, may both have an effect on a patient's appraisal.

Nevertheless, it is often clinically advantageous to plan treatment using a hierarchy of fearful situations.

An Outline of the Fear-Avoidance Model of Chronic Pain

The final strand of current CBT in chronic pain is the application of the fear-avoidance model. Fordyce noted the importance of avoidance, and papers began to explore the relationship between fear, avoidance, and pain in the 1980s. Based on previous work [29,38,49], the development of the fear-avoidance model largely mirrored developments occurring elsewhere, as outlined in Vlaeyen and Linton's initial statement of the model [48]. The basic fear-avoidance conditioning model specific for movement and pain is shown in Fig. 2. Generally, two components are distinguished, a classical component and an operant component. The classical component refers to the process in which a neutral stimulus receives a negative meaning or valence. The person learns to predict events in his/her environment. An injury elicits an automatic response such as muscle tension and sympathetic activation including fear and anxiety. An external

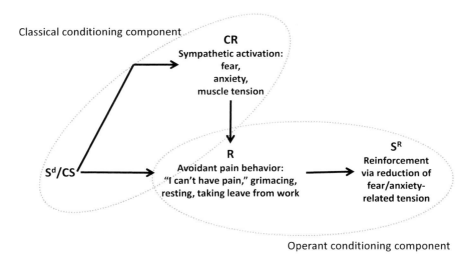

Fig. 2. Classical (Pavlovian) and operant conditioning components in the fear-avoidance model. Redrawn from Vlaeyen and Linton [48].

stimulus may, through classical conditioning, elicit a similar response. Conditioning may take place via direct experience or by information (instructional learning) or even observation (vicarious learning). For example, an individual involved in a traffic accident might develop a fear of driving as a result of the traumatic experience. Likewise, a patient with back pain might develop a fear of lifting after experiencing pain while lifting or after receiving (mis)information that lifting can damage nerves in the spinal cord. The same type of fear can also develop if an individual witnesses someone else having an acute pain attack as a result of lifting. When the stimulus, which precedes the noxious or painful experience, begins to predict the pain, avoidance learning begins. The discriminative stimulus takes on negative valence, which activates muscle reactivity and fear and anxiety itself. Avoiding the threatening situation, as illustrated in Fig. 2, is reinforced by reductions in pain, fear, tension, and anxiety. Once established, avoidance behavior is extremely resistant to extinction. This is because successful avoidance prevents the individual from coming into contact with the actual (nonharmful) consequence of the threatening situation. Moreover, fear will return whenever the avoidance behavior cannot be carried out.

The fear-avoidance model was introduced as a way to describe how pain disability, affective distress, and physical disuse develop as a result of learning protective behaviors such as escape/avoidance behaviors, subtle safety behaviors, and selective attention elicited by pain-related stimuli. In contrast to the conceptualization of chronic pain espoused in the general model of CBT, the fear-avoidance model is relatively specific. In its primary form, it applies to a subgroup of patients who express fears that engaging in specified movements will result in catastrophic consequences. The model provides both an account of how, for this group of patients, a range of unwanted consequences associated with chronic pain can arise and be maintained (i.e., it has an etiological component), and it also predicts how this situation might be altered therapeutically. A diagrammatic representation of this model is shown in Fig. 3.

This more cognitively oriented model of pain-related fear serves as a heuristic aid and incorporates several findings from the literature concerning the role of fear avoidance in the development of musculoskeletal pain problems. It postulates two opposing behavioral responses, confrontation and avoidance, and presents possible pathways by which injured patients get caught in a spiral of increasing avoidance, disability, and pain. The model predicts several ways in which pain-related fear can lead to disability as follows: (1) negative appraisals regarding pain and its consequences, such as catastrophic thinking, are considered a potential precursor for pain-related fear; (2) fear is characterized by escape and avoidance behaviors, the immediate consequences of which are that daily activities (expected to produce pain) are not accomplished, and avoidance of daily activities results in functional disability; (3) because avoidance behaviors occur in anticipation of pain rather than in response to pain, these behaviors may persist because there are fewer opportunities to correct the (wrongful) expectancies and beliefs of pain as a signal of threat to physical integrity; (4) longstanding avoidance and physical inactivity has a detrimental effect on the musculoskeletal and cardiovascular systems, leading to the so-called disuse syndrome, which can further worsen the pain problem. In addition, avoidance also means the withdrawal from essential reinforcers, increasing mood disturbances such as irritability, frustration, and depression. Both depression and disuse are known to be associated

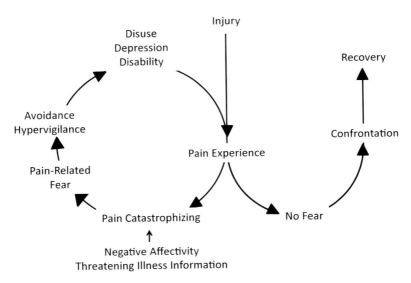

Fig. 3. Simple schematic representation of the fear-avoidance model. Redrawn from Vlaeyen and Linton [48].

with decreased pain tolerance, and hence they might promote the painful experience. From a cognitive-behavioral perspective, there are a number of additional predictions that can be derived from this model; (5) just as with other forms of fear and anxiety, pain-related fear interferes with cognitive functioning. Fearful patients will attend more to possible signals of threat (hypervigilance) and will be less able to shift attention away from pain-related information. This will be at the expense of other tasks including actively coping with problems of daily life; (6) pain-related fear will be associated with increased psychophysiological reactivity when the individual is confronted with situations that are appraised as dangerous.

In essence, the fear-avoidance model simply states that in some circumstances, an individual associates making specific movements with harmful consequences. These movements are appraised as threatening and provoke a state of fear (subjectively unpleasant arousal). This fear might be mitigated by avoiding the activity and also by engaging in safety behavior. Thus, individuals who believe that bending might cause back damage, for example disk prolapse, will avoid a range of bending movements. They might also develop several other behaviors that provide them with a sense of safety, for example wearing a rigid back support or guarding their movement by holding their back when making movements that approximate the feared ones. Treatment proceeds by having patients test the validity of their appraisals by engaging in the very behavior of which they are frightened. In many regards, the fear-avoidance model captures the essence of CBT, which is the careful formulation of an individual's problem followed by treatment devised to test their assumptions and alternative ways of responding via individualized behavioral experiments [5].

The Practice of Cognitive-Behavioral Therapy

Before we examine the fear-avoidance model and treatment implications in more detail (Chapter 2), we briefly consider some essential features of CBT that are not related to treatments for specific problems. Given the variety of contemporary psychological approaches to chronic pain that are generally regarded as representative of CBT, is it possible to provide a definition of CBT that is not a list of techniques? Can we regard it as a unified treatment in any sense? And where does the specific fear-avoidance model fit in the overall picture? In this section, we briefly discuss what might be termed the "meta" attributes of CBT because they provide a framework for understanding the essential components of the fear-avoidance model and its associated treatment protocol. Various definitions of CBT can be found in textbooks, self-help guides and manuals, and in the extensive online resources available. Most of these include the following features (the following list was developed according to the British Association for Behavioural & Cognitive Psychotherapies definition [http://www.babcp.com/Public/What_is_CBT.aspx]):

1) *Cognitive-behavioral therapy interventions are psychological approaches based on scientific principles that research has shown to be effective for a wide range of problems.* There are two elements of this statement. The first is that the interventions are developed from principles derived from primary research on fundamental psychological processes in the laboratory. The second is that implementation of the treatment has been evaluated in a scientifically controlled trial. Whereas both of these statements are true to some extent, many interventions have been initially based on acute clinical observations and case studies followed later by more extensive scientific exploration. Similarly, given the current rapid rate at which CBT is developing, the evidence for treatment effectiveness lags behind the range of problems to which CBT has been applied. With regard to the fear-avoidance model, we will describe both the fundamental research (Chapter 2) on which treatment is based, and in Chapter 6, we will review the available evidence evaluating the implementation of treatment. One aim of this book is to encourage active evaluation of the treatment in routine clinical practice.

2) *Cognitive-behavioral therapy is a collaborative experience based on a strong therapeutic alliance.* Therapeutic alliance refers to the relationship between the patient and the therapist. Various schools of psychotherapy have construed the alliance as being more or less essential to the effectiveness of the treatment. Although a strong therapeutic alliance is seen as an essential component of CBT, unlike psychotherapies derived from psychodynamic or humanistic precepts, it is not the treatment *per se.* A strong therapeutic alliance is necessary for many reasons. For example, the patient must trust the therapist sufficiently to disclose the nature of his/her problem and feel confident enough to experiment with new ways of

behaving that appear potentially threatening and contrary to their needs. The most important focus of the relationship is to facilitate the development of a *shared* view of the patient's problem. It is important that the patient takes ownership of his/her problem and the proposed therapeutic remedy.

3) *Therapy in CBT is centered on the individual case conceptualization (also known as a "case formulation"), which is shared with the patient.* One significant part of the assessment process is to facilitate the development of a shared view of the patient's problem that identifies and frames the problem in terms of the relationship between thoughts, feelings, and behavior. Although within therapy the attention is to the patient's experience, the skill of the therapist is to map the patient's experience onto a validated model of the problem. Specific models for a range of problems, for example social phobia, panic disorder, and depression, have been developed and subjected to considerable research scrutiny. We will address this issue with respect to chronic pain in Chapter 2.

4) *Cognitive-behavioral therapy usually focuses on difficulties in the here and now rather than attending in detail to past relationships and trauma.* Although practitioners of CBT are not disinterested in the etiology of the condition or the background for their clients condition, for the most part the focus in assessment and treatment is on the context (events, thoughts, and behaviors) that are functionally related to the current manifestation of the problem.

5) *Cognitive-behavioral therapy aims to identify personalized and time-limited therapy goals and strategies that are continually monitored and evaluated.* The three elements in this component are central to the implementation of the fear-avoidance model. One key feature of the model is that although the psychological processes underlying the development of avoidance are quite general, the expression of these principles may be quite different across individuals. This is captured in the phrase "generality of process but specificity of content" [44]. It is therefore essential that each patient's problem be considered in a personalized manner. This approach to assessment is described in Chapters 3 and 4, in which despite the use of a uniform set of assessment tools, the emphasis is on the assessment, leading to a highly personalized formulation. Treatment is also time limited. As with any new treatment, determining how long one should

persist with a treatment before reviewing and perhaps terminating it is a largely empirical exercise. With regard to the fear-avoidance model, we have had two contrasting experiences. When testing the model in patients with musculoskeletal pain, we have observed therapeutic changes during the first or second treatment session. However, when extending the treatment to patients with type I chronic regional pain syndrome (CRPS-I), the initial sessions often provoke a worsening of pain, and improvement is not observed for several sessions. These observations appear to be quite robust (Chapter 6). Finally, we advocate careful monitoring and evaluation of treatment for each clinical case. Chapter 6 will describe how this has been achieved in a series of single case studies and where the measures used in these studies are available for routine clinical treatment.

6) *Cognitive-behavioral therapy is inherently empowering.* A significant aim of CBT is to focus on the patient acquiring specific psychological and practical skills. In most cases, this is centered on the patient reflecting on and exploring the meaning that they attribute to events and situations and to their own behavior. The patient is given the opportunity, via discussion and specific behavioral change exercises, to re-evaluate meanings. Treatment aims to enable the patient to tackle their problem by harnessing their own resources, and most treatments inculcate this via planned homework assignments carried out between treatment sessions. The key aim is to facilitate the patient's attribution of therapeutic gain as a consequence of their own efforts, in collaboration with the therapist, rather than to any special quality of the therapist that is outside of their control.

References

[1]   Austin DW, Richards JC. The catastrophic misinterpretation model of panic disorder. Behav Res Ther 2001;39:1277–91.
[2]   Barlow DH. A psychological model of panic. In: Shaw BF, Segal ZV, Vallis TM, Cashman F, editors. Anxiety disorders: psychological and biological perspectives. New York: Plenum Press; 1987.
[3]   Beck AT, Emery G, Greenberg RL. Anxiety disorders and phobias: a cognitive perspective. New York: Basic Books; 1985.
[4]   Beck AT, Rush AJ, Shaw BF, Greenberg RL. Cognitive therapy of depression. New York: Guilford Press; 1979.
[5]   Bennett-Levy J, Butler G, Fennell M, Hackman A, Mueller M, Westbrook D. Oxford guide to behavioural experiments in cognitive therapy. Oxford: Oxford University Press; 2004.
[6]   Bishop SR, Lau M, Shapiro S, Carlson L, Anderson ND, Carmody J, Segal ZV, Abbey S, Speca M, Velting D, Devins G. Mindfulness: a proposed operational definition. Clin Psychol Sci Pract 2004;11:230–41.

[7]   Boudewyns PA, Shipley RH. Flooding and implosive therapy: direct therapeutic exposure in clinical practice. New York: Plenum Press; 1983.
[8]   Brantley J. Mindfulness-based stress reduction. In: Orisllo SM, Roemer L, editors. Acceptance and mindfulness-based approaches to anxiety conceptualization and treatment. New York: Springer; 2005. p. 131–45.
[9]   Budzynski TH, Stoyva JM, Adler CS, Mullaney D. EMG biofeedback and tension headache: a controlled outcome study. Psychosom Med 1973;35:484–96.
[10] Butler AC, Chapman JE, Forman EM, Beck AT. The empirical status of cognitive-behavioral therapy: a review of meta-analyses. Clin Psychol Rev 2006;26:17–31.
[11] Clark DM. A cognitive approach to panic. Behav Res Ther 1986;24:461–70.
[12] Clark DM, Wells A. A cognitive model of social phobia. In: Heimberg RG, Liebowitz MM, Hope D, Scheier F, editors. Social phobia: diagnosis, assessment, and treatment. New York: Guilford; 1995. p. 69–93.
[13] Dahl J, Wilson KG, Nilsson A. Acceptance and commitment therapy and the treatment of persons at risk for long-term disability resulting from stress and pain symptoms: a preliminary randomized trial. Behav Ther 2004;35:785–801.
[14] Dimidjian S, Barrera M, Jr., Martell C, Munoz RF, Lewinsohn PM. The origins and current status of behavioral activation treatments for depression. Annu Rev Clin Psychol 2011;7:1–38.
[15] Ekers D, Richards D, Gilbody S. A meta-analysis of randomized trials of behavioural treatment of depression. Psychol Med 2008;38:611–23.
[16] Ellenberger HF. The discovery of the unconscious: the history and evolution of dynamic psychiatry. New York: Basic Books; 1970.
[17] Erwin E. Behavior therapy: scientific, philosophical and moral foundations. Cambridge: Cambridge University Press; 1978.
[18] Ferster CB. A functional analysis of depression. Am Psychol 1973;28:857–70.
[19] Fordyce WE. Behavioral methods for chronic pain and illness. St Louis: Mosby; 1976.
[20] Fordyce WE, Fowler R, Lehmann J, DeLateur B. Some implications of learning in problems of chronic pain. J Chron Dis 1968;21:179–90.
[21] Gatchel RJ, Peng YB, Peters ML, Fuchs PN, Turk DC. The biopsychosocial approach to chronic pain: scientific advances and future directions. Psychol Bull 2007;133:581–624.
[22] Hayes SC, Barnes-Holmes D, Roche B. Relational frame theory: a post-Skinnerian account of human language and cognition. New York: Kluwer; 2001.
[23] Holmes EA, Mathews A. Mental imagery in emotion and emotional disorders. Clin Psychol Rev 2010;30:349–62.
[24] Jacobson NS, Martell CR, Dimidjian S. Behavioural activation treatment for depression: returning to contextual roots. Clin Psychol Sci Pract 2001;8:255–70.
[25] Kabat-Zinn J. An outpatient program in behavioral medicine for chronic pain patients based on the practice of mindfulness meditation: theoretical considerations and preliminary results. Gen Hosp Psychiatry 1982;4:33–47.
[26] Kazdin AE, Wilcoxon LA. Systematic desensitization and nonspecific treatment effects: a methodological evaluation. Psychol Bull 1976;83:729–58.
[27] Keefe FJ, Beaupré PM, Gil KM, Rumble ME, Aspnes AK. Group therapy with patients with chronic pain. In: Turk DC, Gatchel RJ, editors. Psychological approaches to pain management: a practitioner's handbook. New York: Guilford Press; 2002. p. 234–55.
[28] Lazarus RS, Folkman S. Stress, appraisal and coping. New York: Springer; 1984.
[29] Lethem J, Slade PD, Troup JD, Bentley G. Outline of a fear-avoidance model of exaggerated pain perception: I. Behav Res Ther 1983;21:401–8.
[30] Mahoney MJ, Thoresen CE. Self-control: power to the person. Monterey: Brooks/Cole; 1974.
[31] Martell C, Addis M, Jacobson N. Depression in context. Strategies for guided action. New York: Norton; 2001.
[32] McCracken LM. Contextual cognitive-behavioral therapy for chronic pain. Progress in pain research and management, vol. 33. Seattle: IASP Press; 2005.
[33] Miller NE. Biofeedback and visceral learning. Annu Rev Psychol 1978;28:373–404.
[34] Morley S. Efficacy and effectiveness of cognitive behaviour therapy for chronic pain: progress and some challenges. Pain 2011;152:S99–106.
[35] Morley S, Eccleston C. Cognitive-behaviour therapy for chronic pain in adults. In: Wilson P, Jensen T, Watson PJ, Haythornthwaite JA, Justins DM, editors. Textbook of clinical pain management: chronic pain, vol. 2. London: Hodder Stoughton; 2008.

24 J.W.S. Vlaeyen et al.

[36] Morone NE, Greco CM, Weiner DK. Mindfulness meditation for the treatment of chronic low back pain in older adults: a randomized controlled pilot study. Pain 2008;134:310–9.
[37] Naylor MR, Keefe FJ, Brigidi B, Naud S, Helzer JE. Therapeutic Interactive Voice Response for chronic pain reduction and relapse prevention. Pain 2008;134:335–45.
[38] Philips HC. Avoidance behaviour and its role in sustaining chronic pain. Behav Res Ther 1987;25:273–9.
[39] Rachman S. Fear and courage. New York: W.H. Freeman & Company; 1990.
[40] Rachman S. Joseph Wolpe (1915–1997): Obituary. Amer Psychol 2000;55:431–2.
[41] Rachman S. Psychological treatment of anxiety: The evolution of behavior therapy and cognitive behavior therapy. Ann Rev Clin Psychol 2009;5:97–119.
[42] Sarafino EP. Behavior modification: principles of behavior change. Long Grove, Illinois: Waveland Press; 2001.
[43] Schutze R, Rees C, Preece M, Schutze M. Low mindfulness predicts pain catastrophizing in a fear-avoidance model of chronic pain. Pain 2011;148:120–7.
[44] Shapiro MB. The requirements and implications of a systematic science of psychopathology. Bull Brit Psychol Soc 1975;28:149–55.
[45] Skinner BF. The behavior of organisms: an experimental analysis. Oxford: Appleton-Century; 1938.
[46] Thorn BE. Cognitive therapy for chronic pain. New York: Guilford Press; 2004.
[47] Turk DC, Meichenbaum D, Genest M. Pain and behavioral medicine: a cognitive-behavioral perspective. New York: Guilford Press; 1983.
[48] Vlaeyen JW, Linton SJ. Fear-avoidance and its consequences in chronic musculoskeletal pain: a state of the art. Pain 2000;85:317–32.
[49] Waddell G, Newton M, Henderson I, Somerville D, Main CJ. A fear-avoidance beliefs questionnaire (FABQ) and the role of fear-avoidance beliefs in chronic low-back-pain and disability. Pain 1993;52:157–68.
[50] Wampold BE, Minami T, Baskin TW, CallenTierney S. A meta-(re) analysis of the effects of cognitive therapy versus 'other therapies' for depression. J Affect Disord 2002;68:159–65.
[51] Watson JB, Rayner R. Conditioned emotional reactions. J Exp Psychol 1920;3:1–14.
[52] Watts FN. Habituation model of systematic desensitization. Psychol Bull 1979;86:627–37.
[53] Williams AC. Cognitive-behavioural pain management: lessons learned. In: McQuay H, Kalso EA, Moore RA, editors. Systematic reviews in pain research: methodology refined. Seattle: IASP Press; 2008. p. 275–84.
[54] Wolpe J. Psychotherapy by reciprocal inhibition. Stanford, CA: Stanford University Press; 1958.
[55] Zautra AJ, Davis MC, Reich JW, Nicassio P, Tennen H, Finan P, Kratz A, Parrish B, Irwin MR. Comparison of cognitive behavioral and mindfulness meditation interventions on adaptation to rheumatoid arthritis for patients with and without history of recurrent depression. J Consult Clin Psychol 2008;76:408–21.

Pain-Related Fear in Chronic Pain 2

In this chapter, we examine the fear-avoidance model in more detail. We describe the components of the model, briefly outline the theoretical basis for the model, and consider some of the evidence. This chapter covers the following topics: we will begin this chapter with the basic assumption that pain is a phylogenetically based aversive stimulus, eliciting protective behavior, and that adaptation to painful events occurs via verbal, observational, and experiential learning. We will lay out the differences among exteroceptive, proprioceptive, and interoceptive conditioned stimuli that might signal the occurrence of pain, and highlight the role of pain predictability and the distinction between fear of pain and pain anxiety. We subsequently review the evidence that pain-related fear may act as a significant vulnerability factor for the inception of acute pain and as a maintaining factor for the development of chronic pain. We also will review the literature on the role of catastrophic (mis)interpretations and their relation to pain-related fear. These are the central elements of the fear-avoidance model that were outlined in the previous chapter. This chapter reflects an accumulating body of evidence that has been gathered during the past 10 years, supporting the major assumptions of the fear-avoidance model [2,3,11,45,77,85]. Despite the considerable progress made in the understanding of the role of fear in the development of chronic pain, we also identify gaps in our current knowledge and point to critical theoretical and clinical issues that may guide future clinical research and practice in this area.

Fear, Anxiety, and the Threat of Pain

Pain is an unconditioned stimulus (US) that is considered a biologically relevant signal urging the organism to escape from a dangerous situation, facilitating survival. Pain has some features that are distinct from many other stimuli. First, it is one of those rare stimuli that cannot be shared with others [4]. Second, pain has at least two dimensions, a sensory-discriminative one and an affective-motivational one, reflecting the complex nature of pain perception [59]. Third, the implications of pain are ambiguous. Whereas it is undeniably needed for survival in acute situations and is advantageous, pain can become an important element of suffering when it persists and becomes chronic. In the remainder of this chapter, we will especially focus on the psychological mechanism that may be responsible for the latter situation.

As a biologically relevant stimulus, an acute painful stimulus elicits unlearned responses, often referred to as "reflexes," which are based on genetic endowment. René Descartes described pain as a "reflex of the mind upon damaging stimuli in the periphery of the body, the same way as a church bell [rings] when its connecting ropes are being pulled." But besides automatic withdrawal from the painful stimulus, other defensive responses are engaged during an encounter with a harmful event. Typical unconditioned responses include the orientation of attention to the stimulus, physiological arousal, rapid behavioral withdrawal from the stimulus, and nonverbal expressions such as facial flinching. We will briefly describe each of them in more detail later. Of interest is that these defensive responses are quite similar to those that we recognize when we infer fear or anxiety, two related but functionally distinct concepts. The difference between fear and anxiety depends on imminence of the threat.

Fear refers to the emotional reaction to a specific, identifiable, and immediate threat, such as a dangerous animal or an injury [63]. Fear may protect the individual from impending danger because it instigates defensive behaviors associated with the fight or flight (escape) response.

Sometimes, individuals who rate themselves as being fearful display little or no fear when exposed to fearful stimuli. One of the putative reasons for this discordance is that contextual variables may play a role as well [52]. For example, the availability of safety signals that indicate a period of release from the aversive event may weaken the avoidance response, whereas excessive avoidance behaviors occur when the individual overestimates the level of threat. Defensive escape behaviors reduce fear levels in the short term, although they may strengthen the fear in the long term. They may prevent disconfirmation of an individual's beliefs and sometimes make the feared outcome more likely to occur. Intense, but irrational, fears are called "phobias."

In contrast to fear, *anxiety* is a future-oriented affective state in which the source of threat is not yet detected but is anticipated; it is more elusive, without a clear focus, and hence more uncertain. Anxiety is said to occur when there is no distinct or observable cue that predicts the occurrence of the aversive event. Hence, there is a continued absence of safety, a result of which more long-lasting contextual stimuli elicit preventive responding [30,66]. Furthermore, whereas fear motivates the individual to engage immediately in defensive behaviors, such as escape, anxiety is associated with preventive behaviors, including hypervigilance, catastrophic worry, and avoidance behavior. Hypervigilance occurs when the individual engages in scanning the environment for potential sources of threat and then selectively attends to threat-related rather than neutral stimuli. Hypervigilance broadens the attention before the detection of threat stimuli and narrows the attention in the presence of such stimuli [16]. Consistent with the preparatory function of anxiety, catastrophic worry and related problem-solving emerge as typical features, with the intended function of resolving experienced uncertainty. Avoidance of possible sources of threat is also one of these preparatory behaviors.

Physiological, Behavioral, and Cognitive Responses to Pain

In this section, we summarize current knowledge regarding each of the typical unconditioned responses to pain. We consider pain-related defensive responses a subclass of those that are considered fear-related.

Physiological Arousal

When individuals are exposed to anxiety-eliciting stimuli, a number of changes occur in the autonomic nervous system including in skin conductance levels, muscular reactivity, and heart rate [49]. Extensive research by Flor and colleagues [19,20,22] suggests that psychophysiological responses to chronic pain are symptom specific and stress related. For example, compared to healthy control subjects, patients with chronic low back pain show elevated reactivity of the paralumbar musculature when confronted with a personally relevant stressor and not with stressors in general. Similar elevations were found in symptom-specific body musculature for patients with tension headache (musculus frontalis) and patients with temporomandibular pain dysfunction (musculus masseter). This response stereotypically appears to be limited to the muscular system and is not observed in measures of the autonomic system. Similarly, for the subgroup of patients with chronic low back pain with substantial pain-related fear, one can predict elevated paraspinal electromyographic (EMG) activity to occur when these patients are confronted with movements that they believe are harmful. This muscular reactivity to stress may further maintain the pain problem. Psychophysiological reactivity in fearful patients with chronic low back pain was studied in an experiment in which the participants were presented a video recording including a neutral situation (a nature documentary) followed by a physical activity being performed rigorously by a stooge in the guise of a patient [87]. The patients remained seated during the 6-minute video exposure and were instructed to watch carefully because they would be asked to perform the same activity at the end of the video presentation. Electromyographic activity from four muscles (bilateral lower paraspinal muscles and tibialis anterior muscles) was recorded continuously. The results were partly as predicted and partly surprising. Although self-reported subjective tension during the activity exposure increased relative to that during the nature documentary in the fearful patients with chronic low back pain, there was a decrease in muscular reactivity during both stimuli. However, this decrease was significantly less in fearful patients, who remained at about the same level of reactivity. It seemed that contextual fear caused by the experimental setup produced increased muscular reactivity during baseline. The nonfearful patients readily habituated, while the fearful patients did not. As predicted, the reactivity was symptom specific; only the reactivity of the left erector spinae was predicted by fear of movement/(re)injury. Extending the diathesis-stress model described by Flor and colleagues [19,20], the reactivity of muscles other than the paraspinal muscles (tibialis anterior muscles) was also influenced by pain-related fear but only in the subgroup of patients reporting high on a measure of negative affectivity. In addition, change in lower paraspinal EMG activity predicted subsequent pain reporting during a lifting task in the expected direction; fewer decreases in EMG activity predicted higher pain ratings. Although these results are in line with the studies of Flor and colleagues, further studies are needed to fully understand the consequences of this muscular reactivity. Given the proliferation of neuroimaging techniques in the past decades, scientific attention has shifted from peripheral psychophysiology to cortical reorganization in response to pain [17,18,21].

Escape, Avoidance, and Safety-Seeking Behavior

When an individual finds oneself in an aversive situation, escape from the situation is one of the first protective behaviors to occur. When learning has taken place, and the individual can predict more or less when and where the aversive event might happen, avoidance behavior occurs. Avoidance refers to behavior aimed at postponing or preventing an aversive situation from occurring [40]. When total avoidance is impossible, and escape undesirable, the patient may engage in what are called "safety-seeking behaviors" [69,75]. These are behavioral avoidance strategies that may be used to reduce the anticipated threat when in an aversive situation. Usually, these rather subtle behaviors are logically related to certain rules about how the situation can be handled in a safe way. For example, a patient might have the rule, "I'll make sure that I don't lean forward when I'm holding something heavy because that might break my spine." Whereas in the case of chronic pain it is not possible to avoid the pain, it is possible to avoid the perceived threat, in this case the activities assumed to increase pain or (re)injury. Avoidance behavior might thus be reflected in submaximal performance of activities related to fear. Leeuw and colleagues [45] presented an overview of studies demonstrating that fearful patients with chronic low back pain performed less well on behavioral performance tasks compared to nonfearful patients, pointing to possible withdrawal and thus partial or delayed escape from these tasks. A number of more recent studies also support this assumption. For example, pain-related fear is shown to be associated with decreased walking speed, weakened muscle strength, and diminished performance on physical tasks [74,76,88]. Although there are many studies showing a strong relationship between self-reported avoidance behavior and physical performance, studies measuring actual avoidance behavior are rather scarce. Similarly, there is almost no research available that sheds light on the engagement in subtle safety-seeking behaviors (e.g., not leaning forward while holding a weight for fear of breaking the spine) by patients with chronic pain. As an exception, Tang and colleagues [75] examined the effect of health anxiety on the use of safety-seeking behaviors in patients with chronic low back pain. Whereas the researchers found no differences in the display of overt pain behaviors between patient and healthy control groups, the patient group with highest level of health anxiety deployed a greater number of safety-seeking behaviors than those with low health anxiety or the control group.

The presence of safety-seeking behaviors has important implications for any treatment based on exposure because the rationale for the treatment is that it is only when avoidance is prevented that the patient will learn that the predicted aversive outcome does not occur. However, there is some controversy regarding the deleterious effects of the use of safety-seeking behaviors during exposure treatment for fear-based disorders [62,64]. Some findings suggest that safety-seeking behaviors maintain fear levels because individuals maintain their expectation that an aversive stimulus will follow the conditioned stimulus when no safety behavior is deployed [35,50]. Others claim that the judicious use of safety-seeking behaviors may enhance the extinction of fear, especially in highly anxious patients and at the start of treatment [64]. The effects of safety-seeking behaviors during exposure for pain-related fear still warrant systematic examination.

Cognitive Responses
Attentional Processes

In their seminal article, Eccleston and Crombez captured a central feature of pain, expressing one of its major effects as follows: "Pain demands attention, and interrupts on-going activities even in situations where the current concern of the individual is not related to pain" [13]. Research has revealed that the interruptive quality of pain is determined by the following several parameters: its intensity, novelty, unpredictability, and threat value. Pain may also become the focus of attention because of its immediate relevance for the current goals of the individual. There are many examples in which the processing of pain-related information has priority and has immediate relevance for the goal of the individual. Indeed, in laboratory settings it is almost impossible to find a task that will be able to compete with pain for attentional resources. Outside of the laboratory, anecdotal evidence suggests that it is only when a person is engaged in highly arousing activities, such as competitive sports or life-threatening situations, that pain fails to interrupt conscious experience and behavior. Under most conditions, attention is automatically shifted to pain or cues for pain and, once detected, attention dwells on the pain and is difficult to disengage from it [80,81]. Selective attention to pain is largely automatic and emerges when pain has a high threat value to the individual. It is an unintentional and efficient process that occurs when the individual's current concern is to escape or avoid pain. Evidence shows that it can be controlled, but that control is far from optimal and not without cost. Studies have revealed that attempts to suppress pain or fear may prove futile and may lead to a paradoxical increase in pain or anxious thoughts once attempts to suppress it are stopped [53].

Executive Control

Individuals are able to modify their thoughts and actions via a collection of interrelated abilities known as "executive control." There is evidence that individuals with chronic pain also show deficits in various aspects of cognitive control, such as prospective memory [47], memory updating, flexible task-switching, and task inhibition [71]. Also, pain is known to interrupt the performance of ongoing tasks, and this may be more so in individuals who perceive pain as more threatening [10]. Given that both pain and negative emotions influence cognitive control, patients experiencing pain-related fear are especially at risk for having their executive control functions compromised. An unresolved issue here is what the causal relations are between pain, fear, and cognitive dysfunction.

Pain Catastrophizing

The term "catastrophizing" was first coined by Ellis [16] for the process in which anxious patients dwell on the most extreme negative consequences conceivable. Pain catastrophizing is best conceived as the process during which pain is interpreted as being extremely threatening [67,73]. Pain catastrophizing has consistently been associated with pain disability in patients with pain [57,72,79], as well as in the general population [68]. For example, Sullivan and colleagues [73] provided support for the hypothesis that a patient's level of pain catastrophizing at one point in time is related to subsequent activity intolerance, thereby supporting the notion that catastrophizing predicts future behavior and is not simply a correlate of the patient's current condition. In addition to its association with disability, pain catastrophizing is related to intensified pain in various pain conditions [60]. However, all of these studies are correlational, and no firm causal inferences may be made. One study experimentally manipulated the meaning assigned to a painful stimulus and examined its influence on the pain experience [1]. Healthy volunteers who were led to believe that a cold metal bar applied to the back of the neck was hot rated it as more painful and ascribed more damaging properties to it than other healthy volunteers who were led to believe that the same bar was cold. The damaging interpretation mediated the relationship between the experimental manipulation and the pain experienced. Prospective studies further demonstrated that greater initial levels of pain catastrophizing were related to higher pain intensity during a subsequent painful procedure [14,56], to postoperative pain [41,55], and to long-term adjustment to lower-limb amputation and phantom limb pain [33]. In addition, several studies examining the mediating role of catastrophizing have shown that treatment gains at follow-up are predicted by decreases in catastrophizing during treatment [78]. There is also some evidence that pain catastrophizing might be considered a precursor of pain-related fear. For example, Leeuw and colleagues [46] demonstrated that in low back pain sufferers in the general population, pain catastrophizing was related to pain-related fear 6 months later, even after accounting for other contributing variables such as the initial level of pain-related fear [46]. In another study, the initial level of pain catastrophizing was related to subsequent increases in distress during internal atrial cardioversion, a procedure in which shock is applied to the heart to convert an abnormal rhythm to a normal, regular rhythm [86].

The Consequences of Pain-Related Fear: Associative Learning

Adaptation Through Respondent and Operant Learning

Perhaps one of the most important functions of learning is to predict the occurrence of aversive events in order to take the necessary steps to prevent or mitigate their negative impact. The dominant conceptual framework for exploring learning is associative learning, the term given to theories that account for learning about the relationship between two stimuli or events. The associative learning framework has been applied extensively toward understanding fear and fearful behavior. Here, we briefly describe a modern view of associative learning as the storage of propositional knowledge in memory. Associative learning distinguishes between respondent (also known as "Pavlovian" or "classical" conditioning) learning, which applies to knowledge about the relationship between stimuli, and operant (or "Skinnerian") learning, which concerns knowledge about the relationship between an individual's behavior and a subsequent stimulus or event.

The effects of respondent conditioning are clearly seen when one of the stimuli has no initial influence on behavior (known as the conditioned stimulus, CS) and the other one (the unconditioned stimulus, US) has a reliable capacity to elicit a sequence of responses (the unconditioned response, UR). The central element of respondent conditioning is that neutral stimuli associated with unconditioned aversive stimuli (US) develop fearful qualities and become conditioned fear stimuli (CS), eliciting URs in the absence of the US. According to the theory, the likelihood of fear developing is increased by exposure to high-intensity pain and/or fear situations and by frequent repetitions of the association between the new CS and pain and fear. When objects and situations acquire fear-provoking qualities, they develop motivating properties and elicit conditioned (defensive) responses. For example, neutral visual cues, such as colored dots on a computer screen, may start eliciting fearful responses when associated with painful stimuli (US).

According to the operant learning theory, the likelihood of the occurrence of a behavior is a function of its consequences. The basic principles first introduced by Skinner [70] were applied to pain and illness behaviors by Fordyce and colleagues [23–26]. Specifically, functionally similar behaviors are exhibited more frequently when followed by favorable outcomes (positive reinforcement) or by the removal of unfavorable outcomes (negative reinforcement); the inverse occurs when negative outcomes follow behaviors (positive punishment) or when positive outcomes are removed (negative punishment). Outcomes that can function as reinforcers of pain behaviors include not only the attention provided by significant others and pain reduction, but also the temporary reduction and inhibition of pain-related fear. In the remainder of this chapter, we will focus on respondent learning mechanisms because they have been studied more extensively in the context of fear learning.

Topography of Stimuli

The natures of the CS and the US determine the particular kind of fear or anxiety. On a continuum from "outside" to "inside" the body (the exteroceptive-interoceptive continuum), three types of sensory receptors can be distinguished: *exteroceptors*, *proprioceptors*, and *interoceptors.*

Exteroceptors are situated close to the body surface and are sensitive to mechanical, chemical, thermal, and electromagnetic energy surrounding the organism (reflecting the experience of touch, taste, smell, sound, and vision). Traditionally, experimental human fear conditioning studies have used paradigms with almost exclusively *exteroceptive* (mostly visual) stimuli, probably because they are relatively easy to include in laboratory studies. For example, Bradley and colleagues [7] presented individuals with a visual cue that signaled the presentation of electric shock ("threat") or no shock ("safe"). All participants responded with greater defensive reactivity, including potentiated eye-blink startle, heightened skin conductance, and cardiac deceleration, in the presence of the threat cue compared to the safe cue.

Proprioceptors are sensitive to the orientation and actions of parts of the body in space. Proprioception is restrictively defined as the perception of posture and movement, also referred to as "postural somesthesis" [43]. Likewise, proprioceptive conditioning occurs in fear learning with a proprioceptive stimulus as the CS. This is illustrated in a recent study in which a particular joystick movement (e.g., moving upward, CS+), as opposed to another movement (e.g., moving downward, CS−), was paired with painful shock on the hand. Compared to the condition in which both movements were explicitly not paired with painful shock, the CS+ movement elicited increased eye-blink startle amplitude and slower movement latency responses [51].

Interoceptors are located in the cavities of the body and form the basis for the neural representation of the viscera and the vascular system. Strangely enough, there is little information in the pain literature on interoceptive fear conditioning. Interoceptive cues (e.g., muscle spasms, mild pain, dizziness) can also become a CS. This might be a particular form of fear conditioning that might differentiate the fear of "pain" construct from the fear of "movement" construct. The fear of pain construct might be more relevant for physical complaints in which the musculoskeletal system is less involved [12].

Sources of Propositional Knowledge

From a logical perspective, the relationship among stimuli (respondent learning) or between behavior and subsequent stimuli (operant learning) can be captured in language in the form of propositions such as, "If P happens, then Q occurs" (e.g., "If the bell rings, then food appears," or "If I cry, then social support appears"). Rachman outlined three pathways in which fear might be acquired [61], and these reflect various ways in which propositional knowledge about the relationship between behavior, stimuli, and pain can be acquired. Studies in which with visual cues or movements are used as the CS are examples of learning by direct experience; the person actually experiences the CS-US relationship. In addition, two other (indirect) pathways have been proposed as follows: instructional learning (or transmission of verbal information), the idea that fears can be acquired by hearing or reading threatening information about some object or situation; and observational (or vicarious) learning, by witnessing someone else experiencing frightening events. These three pathways have relevance for understanding why some people acquire pain-related fear and how their subsequent avoidance activity might lead to a cascade of unwanted consequences.

Direct Experience

The direct way to acquire propositional knowledge about pain and other "neutral" stimuli is via direct experience. If a previously neutral movement is followed by increased pain, that particular movement will be avoided in the future [51]. The term "kinesiophobia" is the term first introduced by Kori and colleagues to describe the process in which movements become a CS, signaling pain and the mental representations that go along with it including the risk of (re)injury [44]. Although there are still only a few experimental tests, numerous clinical and descriptive studies have shown that patients reporting increased fear of movement and (re)injury perform worse on different behavioral tests compared to those reporting less pain-related fear. In fact, these are examples in which a proprioceptive stimulus becomes a CS, signaling pain. From a functional perspective, it might be expected that interoceptive stimuli can also act as a CS. Patients may become fearful when feeling moderate pain because they may have experienced that such pain levels usually are followed by increased pain. In the area of respiratory behavior, the inhalation of low doses of carbon dioxide–enriched air usually provokes mild but aversive bodily sensations including breathlessness, heart pounding, and sweating (US). When a negative odor (CS) is added to the carbon dioxide–enriched air, the odor alone can elicit the same aversive bodily sensations after only three trials [82].

Learning Via Verbal Instruction

The presence of language in humans provides the second pathway to learning about the relationship between events and their consequences. The advantage of not having to experience aversive events to learn about them is clearly immeasurable. Laboratory studies provide many examples of instructional learning. The threat value of pain can be experimentally increased via verbal instructions, for example telling participants who are requested to immerse their hand in a cold pressor tank that, "When feeling a tingling sensation in your hand, this may be the first sign of frostbite" [84]. Similarly, threat of painful shock, communicated by verbal instruction, produced higher defensive reactivity (larger blink reflexes and heightened electrodermal activity) in the presence of colored light, which signaled painful shock [7]. Ample information is usually provided verbally by health care providers during their consultation with patients. A number of studies have shown that health care providers with a more biomechanical treatment attitude are more likely to advise activity restrictions, including restrictions on work resumption, to their patients compared to health care providers who hold a more biopsychosocial view on pain [9,37]. Health care providers' advice for patients with chronic pain may vary substantially. A biomechanically oriented health care provider might suggest that all pain-inducing activities be avoided, thereby suggesting a strong CS-US association between activities and damage. On the contrary, health care providers holding a more biopsychosocial orientation might recommend high levels of activity despite continued pain, suggesting no relationship between activities and harm [38,39,63,65,66]. A study from the United Kingdom [6] revealed that the attitudes and beliefs of health care providers were associated with their advice about return to work. Nearly 30% of the respondents reported that they would advise a patient to stay off work, contrary to UK guidelines. This advice was associated with a biomechanical approach. Based on these and similar findings, it has been suggested that the fear-avoidance model be extended to include health care providers' attitudes and fears as important sources of threat information [54].

Observational Learning

There is also an important nonverbal pathway by which an individual might learn about the relationship between pain and activity, observational or vicarious learning [5]. The mere observation of another person in pain can be sufficient to install fear of that particular pain-related stimulus. An important nonverbal source that provides information regarding propositional knowledge is facial expression. From an evolutionary perspective, facial expression has a communicative value because it warns members of a group that the situation is dangerous and that it may inflict bodily harm [32,90]. In an experimental study using two cold pressor tasks with different-colored water, participants reported being more apprehensive toward immersion in cold water after having observed a model displaying painful facial expressions while immersing their hand in the same-colored water. Even during subsequent immersion, more fear was reported with the same-colored water compared to other-colored water associated with relaxed facial expressions by a model [34].

However, the understanding of facial expressions is not always simple because nonverbal cues to emotion are often ambiguous. In such cases, additional information is needed, and this can include the prior experience of the observing individual or additional verbal information. Goubert and colleagues provide an extended review of observational fear learning in chronic pain [29].

Pain-Related Fear as a Vulnerability Factor for the Inception of Acute Low Back Pain

The fear-avoidance model proposes that fear-avoidance beliefs may come into play when an acute pain problem emerges. It therefore appears sensible to assume that fear-avoidance beliefs also exist in pain-free individuals. These beliefs are probably based on previous low back pain experiences, verbal information, observational learning or pre-existing personality traits. For example, pain-free individuals in the general population reported pain-related fear comparable to, or only slightly less than, that of patients with acute or chronic pain [36]. Furthermore, misconceptions, such as those regarding biomedical cause or the presence of unrealistically high expectations regarding medical diagnosis and treatment possibilities for chronic low back pain, are very common in the general population [28]. These fearful beliefs may act as a vulnerability factor for the inception of a new low back pain episode in pain-free individuals. Fearful individuals might be more inclined to misinterpret ambiguous physical sensations as threatening or painful and therefore have an increased likelihood of experiencing pain. There is indeed some evidence that fear-avoidance beliefs heighten the probability of subsequently developing a new pain episode. In a study of pain-free individuals, pain-related fear substantially increased the risk of subsequent inception of low back pain and diminished physical functioning [48]. In addition, in workers who were pain free, a higher risk for future low back pain onset was found for those who catastrophized pain and for those with heightened pain-related fear [83]. Because these studies included participants who were pain free during the past year, it is important to recognize that the included participants were not pain free in the sense that they had never experienced low back pain before. Owing to its high prevalence, it is very likely that these participants had suffered previous low back pain episodes, which might have influenced the initiation of a new episode.

Pain-Related Fear as a Risk Factor for the Development of Chronic Low Back Pain

The evidence that beliefs about the relationship between the harmful nature of activities and avoidance of these activities (fear-avoidance beliefs) might be related to both the inception and continuation of low back pain remains ambiguous. A difference in the stringency of evaluating studies in several reviews of the evidence has resulted in variation in the conclusions drawn. Linton and colleagues [48] concluded that fear-avoidance beliefs were associated with both the inception and continuation of low back pain, whereas others concluded that although psychological factors, such as distress, depressive mood, and somatization, were implicated in the transition to chronic low back pain, there was less evidence for the other psychological factors including pain-related fear. More recently, several studies have investigated pain-related fear during the acute pain phase. In patients with acute low back pain, pain-related fear was found to be associated with diminished participation in activities of daily life, perceived disability, work loss, and diminished performance on a lifting task [31,74]. What is lacking is a test of the dynamic and sequential relationships among these variables. A study of young workers who had no back pain at baseline, but some of whom developed pain at follow-up, revealed that pain-related fear in these pain-free individuals was predictive of disability. In addition, pain-related fear did not predict pain later on but came into play once low back pain was experienced. These results suggest that it is more parsimonious to view pain-related fear as a consequence of pain severity, which does not necessarily imply that its effects are redundant with those of pain severity [27]. Similar findings were reported in a large cohort of female health care workers [39]. Pain-related fear appeared to increase the risk for sickness absence 1 year later, even when controlling for work-related confounding factors. In addition, pain severity moderated the association between pain-related fear and sickness absence. Health care workers who reported high levels of pain-related fear reported more sickness absence when they also reported high pain severity [39]. A prospective sequential analysis of the fear-avoidance model of pain conducted by Wideman and colleagues [89] in patients participating in a pain management program revealed that early changes in catastrophizing, late changes in pain severity, and late changes in fear of movement were significant predictors of return to work, with changes in pain catastrophizing being the more robust independent variable. These authors suggested that this may be due to the inclusion of helplessness items as part of the measure of pain catastrophizing [89]. Moreover, it may well be that interrelations among catastrophizing, fear, and disability might differ for the development of pain-related disability compared to interrelations for the recovery of pain-related disability.

The Object of Fear: Beyond Fear of Movement-Related Pain

Fear of pain and associated avoidance behaviors may not be the only kind of fear associated with chronic pain. Given the debilitating consequences of longstanding avoidance behaviors, patients may present with multiple fears and concerns, including the inability to work (functional), having surgery (health), having to sell the house (financial), and being a burden to family members (social). For patients with chronic pain, another important concern may be social isolation that occurs in response to their diminished participation in daily life. Given that individuals with increased sensitivity to pain also appear to respond more sensitively to social rejection, and that a distress reaction to social rejection is itself associated with higher subsequent pain sensitivity, concerns of social isolation in patients with pain inadvertently increase their pain threshold [15].

Morley and Eccleston [53a] propose to broaden the fear-avoidance model to those areas that possess a possible threat to an individual's identity, using Carver and Scheier's goal-oriented model of self-regulation [8]. Following this theory, a distinction is made between approach goals and avoidance goals. Approach goals are those that the individual is hoping for, whereas avoidance goals consist of situations that have a negative value. According to the goal-oriented model, fear is the emotional reaction to a movement toward an avoidance goal. Although this theoretical framework appears to be a promising avenue for broadening current fear-avoidance models, research efforts have just started. For example, Kindermans and colleagues reported that self-discrepancies between feared and actual selves were predictive of depressive and anxious mood and lower self-reported activity levels [42].

Conclusion

The past decade has seen a surge in the study of the fear of pain in both basic and clinical investigations. The recent literature mainly supports the basic assumptions of the fear-avoidance model, but it also provides greater depth, inspiring future research and novel clinical applications. In particular, the model draws on associative learning, and experimental research provides a fertile ground for future work on the intricacies of its mechanisms. The key idea is that preparatory behaviors are adaptive in decreasing fear in the short term, but that they paradoxically maintain fear levels in the long term. There is ample empirical evidence showing that the level of pain-related fear early on (in acute pain or in healthy individuals) predicts long term disability and distress.

References

[1]   Arntz A, Claassens L. The meaning of pain influences its experienced intensity. Pain 2004;109:20–5.
[2]   Asmundson GJ, Norton GR, Allerdings MD. Fear and avoidance in dysfunctional chronic back pain patients. Pain 1997;69:231–6.
[3]   Asmundson GJG, Vlaeyen JWS, Crombez G. Understanding and treating fear of pain. Oxford: Oxford University Press; 2004.
[4]   Auvray M, Myin E, Spence C. The sensory-discriminative and affective-motivational aspects of pain. Neurosci Biobehav Rev 2009;34:214–23.
[5]   Bandura A. Social cognitive theory. In: Vasta R, editor. Six theories of child development, Vol. 6. Greenwich, CT: JAI Press; 1989. p. 1–60.
[6]   Bishop A, Foster NE, Thomas E, Hay EM. How does the self-reported clinical management of patients with low back pain relate to the attitudes and beliefs of health care practitioners? A survey of UK general practitioners and physiotherapists. Pain 2008;135:187–95.
[7]   Bradley MM, Silakowski T, Lang PJ. Fear of pain and defensive activation. Pain 2008;137:156–63.
[8]   Carver CS, Scheier MF. On the self-regulation of behavior. Cambridge: Cambridge University Press; 1998.
[9]   Coudeyre E, Rannou F, Tubach F, Baron G, Coriat F, Brin S, Revel M, Poiraudeau S. General practitioners' fear-avoidance beliefs influence their management of patients with low back pain. Pain 2006;124:330–7.
[10] Crombez G, Eccleston C, Baeyens F, Eelen P. Attentional disruption is enhanced by the threat of pain. Behav Res Ther 1998b;36:195–204.
[11] Crombez G, Eccleston C, Van Damme S, Vlaeyen JW, Karoly P. The fear avoidance model of chronic pain: the next generation. Clin J Pain 2012; in press.

[12] De Peuter S, Van Diest I, Vansteenwegen D, Van den Bergh O, Vlaeyen JW. Understanding fear of pain in chronic pain: Interoceptive fear conditioning as a novel approach. Eur J Pain 2011;15:889–94.

[13] Eccleston C, Crombez G. Pain demands attention: a cognitive-affective model of the interruptive function of pain. Psychol Bull 1999;125:356–66.

[14] Edwards RR, Fillingim RB, Maixner W, Sigurdsson A, Haythornthwaite J. Catastrophizing predicts changes in thermal pain responses after resolution of acute dental pain. J Pain 2004;5:164–70.

[15] Eisenberger NI, Jarcho JM, Lieberman MD, Naliboff BD. An experimental study of shared sensitivity to physical pain and social rejection. Pain 2006;126:132–8.

[15a] Ellis A. Reason and emotion in psychotherapy. New York: Lyle Stuart; 1962.

[16] Eysenck MW. Anxiety and cognition. A unified theory. Hove: Psychology Press; 1997.

[17] Flor H. The functional organization of the brain in chronic pain. Prog Brain Res 2000;129:313–22.

[18] Flor H. Cortical reorganisation and chronic pain: implications for rehabilitation. J Rehabil Med 2003;41(Suppl):66–72.

[19] Flor H, Birbaumer N, Schugens MM, Lutzenberger W. Symptom-specific psychophysiological responses in chronic pain patients. Psychophysiology 1992;29:452–60.

[20] Flor H, Birbaumer N, Schulte W, Roos R. Stress-related electromyographic responses in patients with chronic temporomandibular pain. Pain 1991;46:145–52.

[21] Flor H, Denke C, Schaefer M, Grusser S. Effect of sensory discrimination training on cortical reorganisation and phantom limb pain. Lancet 2001;357:1763–4.

[22] Flor H, Turk DC. Chronic pain: an integrated biobehavioral approach. Seattle: IASP Press; 2011.

[23] Fordyce WE. Behavioral methods for chronic pain and illness. St. Louis: Mosby; 1976.

[24] Fordyce WE, Fowler RS, Jr., Lehmann JF, DeLateur BJ. Some implications of learning in problems of chronic pain. J Chronic Dis 1968;21:179–90.

[25] Fordyce WE, Fowler RS Jr, Lehmann JF, Delateur BJ, Sand PL, Trieschmann RB. Operant conditioning in the treatment of chronic pain. Arch Phys Med Rehabil 1973;54:399–408.

[26] Fordyce WE, Shelton JL, Dundore DE. The modification of avoidance learning pain behaviors. J Behav Med 1982;5:405–14.

[27] Gheldof EL, Crombez G, Van den Bussche E, Vinck J, Van Nieuwenhuyse A, Moens G, Mairiaux P, Vlaeyen JW. Pain-related fear predicts disability, but not pain severity: a path analytic approach of the fear-avoidance model. Eur J Pain 2010;14:870 e871–9.

[28] Goubert L, Crombez G, De Bourdeaudhuij I. Low back pain, disability and back pain myths in a community sample: prevalence and interrelationships. Eur J Pain 2004;8:385–94.

[29] Goubert L, Vlaeyen JW, Crombez G, Craig KD. Learning about pain from others: an observational learning account. J Pain 2011;12:167–74.

[30] Grillon C. Greater sustained anxiety but not phasic fear in women compared to men. Emotion 2008;8:410–3.

[31] Grotle M, Vollestad NK, Veierod MB, Brox JI. Fear-avoidance beliefs and distress in relation to disability in acute and chronic low back pain. Pain 2004;112:343–52.

[32] Hadjistavropoulos T, Craig KD, Duck S, Cano A, Goubert L, Jackson PL, Mogil JS, Rainville P, Sullivan MJ, Williams AC de C, Vervoort T, Fitzgerald TD. A biopsychosocial formulation of pain communication. Psychol Bull 2011;137:910–39.

[33] Hanley MA, Jensen MP, Ehde DM, Hoffman AJ, Patterson DR, Robinson LR. Psychosocial predictors of long-term adjustment to lower-limb amputation and phantom limb pain. Disabil Rehabil 2004;26:882–93.

[34] Helsen K, Goubert L, Peters ML, Vlaeyen JW. Observational learning and pain-related fear: an experimental study with colored cold pressor tasks. J Pain 2011;12:1230–9.

[35] Hood HK, Antony MM, Koerner N, Monson CM. Effects of safety behaviors on fear reduction during exposure. Behav Res Ther 2010;48:1161–9.

[36] Houben RM, Leeuw M, Vlaeyen JW, Goubert L, Picavet HS. Fear of movement/injury in the general population: factor structure and psychometric properties of an adapted version of the Tampa Scale for Kinesiophobia. J Behav Med 2005:1–10.

[37] Houben RM, Ostelo RW, Vlaeyen JW, Wolters PM, Peters M, Stomp-van den Berg SG. Health care providers' orientations towards common low back pain predict perceived harmfulness of physical activities and recommendations regarding return to normal activity. Eur J Pain 2005;9:173–83.

[38] Houben RMA, Ostelo RWJG, Vlaeyen JWS, Wolters PMJC, Peters M, Stomp-van den Berg SGM. Health care providers' orientations towards common low back pain predict perceived harmfulness of physical activities and recommendations regarding return to normal activity. Eur J Pain 2005;9:173–83.

[39] Jensen JN, Karpatschof B, Labriola M, Albertsen K. Do fear-avoidance beliefs play a role on the association between low back pain and sickness absence? A prospective cohort study among female health care workers. J Occup Environ Med 2010;52:85–90.

[40] Kanfer FH, Phillips JS. Learning foundations of behavior therapy. Oxford, England: John Wiley; 1970.

[41] Khan RS, Ahmed K, Blakeway E, Skapinakis P, Nihoyannopoulos L, Macleod K, Sevdalis N, Ashrafian H, Platt M, Darzi A, Athanasiou T. Catastrophizing: a predictive factor for postoperative pain. Am J Surg 2011;201:122–31.

[42] Kindermans HP, Huijnen IP, Goossens ME, Roelofs J, Verbunt JA, Vlaeyen JW. "Being" in pain: The role of self-discrepancies in the emotional experience and activity patterns of patients with chronic low back pain. Pain 2011;152:403–9.

[43] Konorski J. Integrative activity of the brain. An interdisciplinary approach. Chicago: University of Chicago Press; 1967.

[44] Kori SH, Miller RP, Todd DD. Kinesiophobia: a new view of chronic pain behavior. Pain Manag 1990;Jan/Feb:35–43.

[45] Leeuw M, Goossens ME, Linton SJ, Crombez G, Boersma K, Vlaeyen JW. The fear-avoidance model of musculoskeletal pain: current state of scientific evidence. J Behav Med 2007;30:77–94.

[46] Leeuw M, Houben RM, Severeijns R, Picavet HS, Schouten EG, Vlaeyen JW. Pain-related fear in low back pain: a prospective study in the general population. Eur J Pain 2007;11:256–66.

[47] Ling J, Campbell C, Heffernan TM, Greenough CG. Short-term prospective memory deficits in chronic back pain patients. Psychosom Med 2007;69:144–148.

[48] Linton SJ, Buer N, Vlaeyen JWS, Hellsing AL. Are fear-avoidance beliefs related to the inception of an episode of back pain? A prospective study. Psychol Health 2000;14:1051–9.

[49] Loggia ML, Juneau M, Bushnell MC. Autonomic responses to heat pain: heart rate, skin conductance, and their relation to verbal ratings and stimulus intensity. Pain 2011;152:592–8.

[50] Lovibond PF, Mitchell CJ, Minard E, Brady A, Menzies RG. Safety behaviours preserve threat beliefs: protection from extinction of human fear conditioning by an avoidance response. Behav Res Ther 2009;47:716–20.

[51] Meulders A, Vansteenwegen D, Vlaeyen JWS. The acquisition of fear of movement-related pain and associative learning: a novel pain-relevant human fear conditioning paradigm. Pain 2011;152:2460–9.

[52] Mineka S, Zinbarg R. A contemporary learning theory perspective on the etiology of anxiety disorders: it's not what you thought it was. Am Psychol 2006;61:10–26.

[53] Morley S. Attention management. In: Paice JA, Bell RF, Kalso EA, Soyannwo OA, editors. Cancer pain: from molecules to suffering. Seattle: IASP Press; 2010. p. 245–65.

[53a] Morley S, Eccleston C. The object of fear in pain. In: Asmundson GJ, Vlaeyen J, Crombez G, editors. Understanding and treating fear of pain. Oxford: Oxford University Press; 2004. p. 163.

[54] Ostelo RW, Vlaeyen JW. Attitudes and beliefs of health care providers: extending the fear-avoidance model. Pain 2008;135:3–4.

[55] Papaioannou M, Skapinakis P, Damigos D, Mavreas V, Broumas G, Palgimesi A. The role of catastrophizing in the prediction of postoperative pain. Pain Med 2009;10:1452–9.

[56] Pavlin DJ, Sullivan MJ, Freund PR, Roesen K. Catastrophizing: a risk factor for postsurgical pain. Clin J Pain 2005;21:83–90.

[57] Peters ML, Vlaeyen JW, Weber WE. The joint contribution of physical pathology, pain-related fear and catastrophizing to chronic back pain disability. Pain 2005;113:45–50.

[58] Pincus T, Burton AK, Vogel S, Field AP. A systematic review of psychological factors as predictors of chronicity/disability in prospective cohorts of low back pain. Spine 2002;27:E109–20.

[59] Price DD. Psychological and neural mechanisms of the affective dimension of pain. Science 2000;288:1769–72.

[60] Quartana PJ, Campbell CM, Edwards RR. Pain catastrophizing: a critical review. Expert Rev Neurother 2009;9:745–58.

[61] Rachman S. The conditioning theory of fear-acquisition: a critical examination. Behav Res Ther 1977;15:375–87.

[62] Rachman S. Agoraphobia: a safety-signal perspective. Behav Res Ther 1984;22:59–70.

44   J.W.S Vlaeyen et al.

[63] Rachman S. Anxiety. Hove: Psychology Press; 1998.
[64] Rachman S, Radomsky AS, Shafran R. Safety behaviour: a reconsideration. Behav Res Ther 2008;46:163–73.
[65] Rainville J, Bagnall D, Phalen L. Health care providers' attitudes and beliefs about functional impairments and chronic back pain. Clin J Pain 1995;11:287–95.
[66] Rhudy JL, Meagher MW. Fear and anxiety: divergent effects on human pain thresholds. Pain 2000;84:65–75.
[67] Rosenstiel AK, Keefe FJ. The use of coping strategies in chronic low back pain patients: relationship to patient characteristics and current adjustment. Pain 1983;17:33–44.
[68] Severeijns R, Vlaeyen JW, Van Den Hout MA, Picavet HS. Pain catastrophizing is associated with health indices in musculoskeletal pain: a cross-sectional study in the Dutch community. Health Psychol 2004;23:49–57.
[69] Sharp TJ. The "safety seeking behaviours" construct and its application to chronic pain. Behav Cogn Psychother 2001;29:241–4.
[70] Skinner BF. Science and human behavior. New York: McMillan; 1953.
[71] Solber Nes L, Roach A, Segerstrom SC. Executive functions, self-regulation, and chronic pain: a review. Ann Behav Med 2009;37:173–83.
[72] Sullivan MJ, Lynch ME, Clark AJ. Dimensions of catastrophic thinking associated with pain experience and disability in patients with neuropathic pain conditions. Pain 2005;113:310–5.
[73] Sullivan MJ, Stanish W, Waite H, Sullivan M, Tripp DA. Catastrophizing, pain, and disability in patients with soft-tissue injuries. Pain 1998;77:253–60.
[74] Swinkels-Meewisse IE, Roelofs J, Oostendorp RA, Verbeek AL, Vlaeyen JW. Acute low back pain: pain-related fear and pain catastrophizing influence physical performance and perceived disability. Pain 2006;120:36–43.
[75] Tang NK, Salkovskis PM, Poplavskaya E, Wright KJ, Hanna M, Hester J. Increased use of safety-seeking behaviors in chronic back pain patients with high health anxiety. Behav Res Ther 2007;45:2821–35.
[76] Thomas JS, France CR. Pain-related fear is associated with avoidance of spinal motion during recovery from low back pain. Spine (Phila Pa 1976) 2007;32:E460–6.
[77] Turk DC, Wilson HD. Fear of pain as a prognostic factor in chronic pain: conceptual models, assessment, and treatment implications. Curr Pain Headache Rep 2010;14:88–95.
[78] Turner JA, Holtzman S, Mancl L. Mediators, moderators, and predictors of therapeutic change in cognitive-behavioral therapy for chronic pain. Pain 2007;127:276–86.
[79] Turner JA, Mancl L, Aaron LA. Pain-related catastrophizing: a daily process study. Pain 2004;110:103–11.
[80] Van Damme S, Crombez G, Eccleston C. Retarded disengagement from pain cues: the effects of pain catastrophizing and pain expectancy. Pain 2002;100:111–8.
[81] Van Damme S, Crombez G, Eccleston C. Disengagement from pain: the role of catastrophic thinking about pain. Pain 2004;107:70–6.
[82] Van den Bergh O, Winters W, Devriese S, Van Diest I. Learning subjective health complaints. Scand J Psychol 2002;43:147–52.
[83] Van Nieuwenhuyse A, Somville PR, Crombez G, Burdorf A, Verbeke G, Johannik K, Van den Bergh O, Masschelein R, Mairiaux P, Moens GF. The role of physical workload and pain related fear in the development of low back pain in young workers: evidence from the BelCoBack Study; results after one year of follow up. Occup Environ Med 2006;63:45–52.
[84] Vlaeyen JW, Hanssen M, Goubert L, Vervoort T, Peters M, van Breukelen G, Sullivan MJ, Morley S. Threat of pain influences social context effects on verbal pain report and facial expression. Behav Res Ther 2009;47:774–82.
[85] Vlaeyen JW, Linton SJ. Fear-avoidance model of chronic musculoskeletal pain: 12 years on. Pain 2012;153:1144–7.
[86] Vlaeyen JW, Timmermans C, Rodriguez LM, Crombez G, Van Horne W, Ayers GM, Albert A, Wellens HJ. Catastrophic thinking about pain increases discomfort during internal atrial cardioversion. J Psychosom Res 2004;56:139–44.
[87] Vlaeyen JWS, Seelen HA, Peters M, de Jong P, Aretz E, Beisiegel E, Weber WE. Fear of movement/(re)injury and muscular reactivity in chronic low back pain patients: an experimental investigation. Pain 1999;82:297–304.
[88] Vowles KE, Gross RT. Work-related beliefs about injury and physical capability for work in individuals with chronic pain. Pain 2003;101:291–8.

[89] Wideman TH, Adams H, Sullivan MJ. A prospective sequential analysis of the fear-avoidance model of pain. Pain 2009;145:45–51.
[90] Williams AC. Facial expression of pain: an evolutionary account. Behav Brain Sci 2002;25:439–55; discussion 455–88.

Selection and Assessment

In this chapter, we review the methods we have used to select and assess patients who may be suitable for treatment aimed at fear reduction. We will deal with specific questionnaires, the interview, the establishment of graded hierarchies, and behavioral tests that can be applied to gain sufficient information about the idiosyncratic aspects of pain-related fear responses in patients with chronic musculoskeletal pain.

The fundamental question is: What is the patient afraid of? Or in other words, what is the nature of the perceived threat? An answer to this question is not as simple as it seems. Patients may not view their problem as involving fear at all and may simply see difficulty in performing certain movements or activities. In addition, the specific nature of pain-related fear varies considerably, making an idiosyncratic approach almost indispensable. Most patients fear pain itself. Other patients may fear not so much current pain but pain that will be experienced at a later time, for example, the day after increased physical exercise. Finally, patients may not fear pain itself, but the impending (re)injury and the risk of becoming permanently handicapped. For these patients, pain is seen as a warning signal for a seriously threatening situation. The literature reflects this variety of fear stimuli by discussing measures for the assessment of fear of pain, fear of work and physical activity, and fear of (re)injury as a result of movement.

Pain-Related Fear: Exposure-Based Treatment for Chronic Pain
by Johan W.S. Vlaeyen, Stephen J. Morley, Steven J. Linton, Katja Boersma, and Jeroen de Jong
IASP Press, Seattle, © 2012

Specific Questionnaires to Assess Fear or Anxiety in Relation to Pain

Questionnaires can offer a quick and robust method for the initial screening of potentially suitable patients. In addition, questionnaires are often used to measure the outcome of treatment. We have used them for both of these purposes. Several questionnaires that measure fear of pain-related activity have been developed. The major ones are shown in Table I, which also includes sample items. Generally, these measures can be grouped into three classes as follows: those that measure attitudes about pain, those that measure catastrophizing about pain, and those that measure pain-related fear.

Attitudes About Pain

An early attempt to assess fear of pain is the Pain and Impairment Relationship Scale (PAIRS), developed to study attitudes of patients with chronic pain concerning activity and pain [27]. The scale has 15 items that are rated on a 7-point Likert scale, and it has been found to have good psychometric characteristics. The original study demonstrated that beliefs that activity would increase pain were related to physical impairment. The Survey of Pain Attitudes [15] was developed to assess patients' attitudes toward the following five dimensions of the chronic pain experience: pain control, pain-related disability, medical cures for pain, solicitude of others, and medication for pain. The authors added a further subscale (harm) based on their clinical observations of an association between chronic patients' hesitancy to exercise and the expressed fear of possible injury. In addition to the Disability and Control scales, the Harm scale appeared to independently predict levels of dysfunction. These questionnaires have good psychometric qualities in that they show high internal consistency, good test stability, and indications of validity. They are specifically focused on the central component of the fear-avoidance model, that is, the catastrophic appraisal of the relationship between activity and anticipated harm. Although we have tended not to use these questionnaires, there are occasions (see Chapter 6) where we have taken specific items from the questionnaires to construct a measure for use in a particular study.

Measures of Pain Catastrophizing

The concept of catastrophizing about pain has developed over the past 30 years [33]. An individual's propensity to catastrophize, that is, to generate and ruminate on negative outcomes, is recognized as a key psychological process in their adjustment to ongoing pain. Several measures have also been developed to assess the level at which patients perceive pain as catastrophically threatening.

Cognitive Errors Questionnaire (CEQ) [20]. The CEQ was among the earliest measures developed. It comprises the following four subscales: catastrophizing, overgeneralization, personalization, and selective abstraction, identified in Beck's cognitive model of depression as resulting from fundamental cognitive errors. The CEQ is somewhat different from the other measures because it consists of a number of vignettes followed by a brief statement reflecting a thought. Subjects are asked to rate how similar the cognition is to the thought that they would have in a similar situation. There are two versions, a general one and a version for patients with low back pain. Although the CEQ appears to have reasonable psychometric properties, it has not been widely used in clinical research, and this may be because of the "unwieldiness of the instrument and the length of administration" [7].

Coping Strategies Questionnaire (CSQ) [30]. The CSQ has been widely used since its development in 1983. The CSQ has 42 items rated on a 7-point (0–6) response scale. There are seven 6-item subscales that measure several components of coping and appraisal. One of these assesses catastrophizing. The CSQ has been subjected to several psychometric studies to evaluate its factor structure [8], and it has been widely used in a range of studies. The Catastrophizing scale has been used as a stand-alone measure. Its merits are that it is brief and reasonably reliable, but it has been superseded by two other measures that are slightly longer but have arguably better content validity and psychometric properties.

Pain Cognition List (PCL) [36]. The original PCL [39] comprised 77 items divided into five subscales. Each item presents a specific statement related to pain, for example, "My thoughts are always concentrated on the pain," and the patient is asked to indicate agreement or disagreement on a five-point Likert scale. Items are scored from 1 (totally disagree) to 5 (totally agree), and a sum score is obtained per subscale for

Table I
Questionnaires for assessing components of the fear-avoidance model

Questionnaire	Source	No. Items	Subscales	Sample Item
Pain Attitudes				
PAIRS: Pain and Impairment Relationship Questionnaire	Riley et al. [27]	15	Total	
SOPA: Survey of Pain Attitudes	Jensen et al. [15]	8	Harm	
Pain Catastrophizing				
PCS: Pain Catastrophizing Scale	Sullivan et al. [32]	13	Rumination Amplification Helplessness	I keep thinking about how much it hurt. I grow afraid that the pain will get worse. There's nothing I can do to reduce the intensity of the pain.
PCL: Pain Cognition List	Van Breukelen and Vlaeyen [36]	16	Catastrophizing	
CEQ: Cognitive Error Questionnaire	Lefebvre [20]	24	Catastrophizing Overgeneralization Personalization Selective abstraction	Vignettes (e.g., You have a painful back problem but have continued to work. Although you got quite a bit done today, you quit work a little early because your back was really hurting. You think to yourself, "What a terrible day; it seems like I can't get anything done.")
CSQ: Coping Strategies Questionnaire	Rosenstiel and Keefe [30]	6	Catastrophizing	I feel I can't stand it anymore.

Pain-Related Fear

Measure	Reference		Subscale	Example item
TSK: Tampa Scale for Kinesiophobia (original version)	Miller et al. [23]	17		Pain lets me know when to stop exercising so that I don't injure myself.
TSK-11: Tampa Scale for Kinesiophobia	Roelofs et al. [28]	6	Activity avoidance	I can't do all the things normal people do because it's too easy for me to get injured.
		5	Somatic focus	My body is telling me I have something dangerously wrong.
FABQ: Fear-Avoidance Beliefs Questionnaire	Waddell et al. [41]	4	Physical activity	Physical activity might harm my back.
		6	Work	I cannot do my normal work until my pain is treated.
PASS-20: Pain Anxiety Symptoms Scale	McCracken and Dhingra [21]	20	Fearful appraisals	When pain comes on strong, I think I might become paralyzed or more disabled.
			Cognitive anxiety	Pain sensations are terrifying.
			Physiological anxiety	I get sweaty when in pain.
			Escape/avoidance	I immediately go to bed when I feel severe pain.

each patient. On the basis of factor and content analysis, the list was reduced to 39 items. Thus, a more manageable questionnaire was obtained, consisting of five distinct subscales of varying length (from 4 to 16 items) and internal consistency (Cronbach's α of 0.64 to 0.88, mean item-item correlation of 0.28 to 0.35) and with correlations between subscales ranging from 0.00 to 0.45. Validity of these subscales was supported by the meaningful pattern of correlations with other relevant constructs [38]. The largest is the Pain Catastrophizing subscale, with 16 items. Correlation coefficients of approximately 0.70 occur between this subscale and related measures such as the Catastrophizing scale of the CSQ [30] and Pain Catastrophizing Scale [32].

Pain Catastrophizing Scale (PCS) [32]. Perhaps the most widely used measure, the PCS is a 13-item scale developed for both nonclinical and clinical populations. Subjects reflect on past painful experiences and indicate the degree to which they experienced thoughts or feelings more on a five-point scale (e.g., "I can't seem to keep it out of my mind," or "I feel I can't stand it anymore"). The three-factor structure of the PCS, with the subscales Rumination, Magnification, and Helplessness, has been shown to be robust across diagnoses, cultures, and age groups [5,37].

Pain-Related Fear and Anxiety

Specific fear of pain measures also exist. The Pain Anxiety Symptoms Scale (PASS) [22] was developed to measure anxiety symptoms reflected in the following main conceptual components of anxiety: cognitive anxiety symptoms, escape and avoidance responses, fearful appraisals of pain, and physiologic anxiety symptoms related to pain. Later, a 20-item version was introduced with internally consistent subscales [21]. The validity of the PASS has been supported by positive correlations with measures of anxiety, cognitive errors, depression, and disability. A more recent exploratory factor analysis revealed five factors that could be labeled as follows: catastrophic thoughts, physiological anxiety symptoms, escape/avoidance behaviors, cognitive interference, and coping strategies [18].

The Fear-Avoidance Beliefs Questionnaire (FABQ) [41] focuses on patients' beliefs about how work and physical activity affect their low back pain. The FABQ consists of two scales, fear-avoidance beliefs about physical activity and fear-avoidance beliefs about work, of which the latter is consistently the stronger. The authors found that fear-avoidance beliefs about work are strongly related to daily living disability and work lost in the past year, more so than biomedical variables such as anatomical pattern of pain, time pattern, and severity of pain. However, the FABQ Physical subscale is much stronger in predicting behavioral performance tests [6].

The original version of the Tampa Scale for Kinesiophobia (TSK) [23] was a 17-item questionnaire that aimed to assess fear of (re)injury owing to movement. Each item is provided with a four-point Likert scale, with scoring alternatives ranging from "strongly agree" to "strongly disagree" (coded 1–4, giving a maximum score of 68). Most psychometric research has been carried out with the Dutch version of the TSK, which appears to be sufficiently reliable [28,40]. Several researchers have noted that the psychometric qualities of the scale are affected by some reverse-scored items, and the properties of the scale might be improved by reducing the number of items and restructuring it [12]. Indeed, a recent psychometric analysis supported an 11-item version with two subscales, Activity Avoidance and Somatic Focus [29]. Because of the relatively high intercorrelations among the subscales, the TSK total score can be used as well. The TSK has the advantage that it has been tested in various pain populations and that its factor structure has been shown to be invariable across pain diagnoses and different nationalities. Despite the limitations of the original TSK, we have used it extensively both as a preliminary screening tool and as an outcome measure in the series of studies reported in Chapter 6. The main reason for this decision is that in comparison to the PASS and FABQ, the TSK most closely matches the aspect of pain-related fear that we have focused on in the development of treatment regarding the fear-avoidance model, that is, the relationship between movement and the threat of a harmful outcome.

In summary, several questionnaires for the assessment of pain-related fear are now available, although the validity of some of them needs further exploration. For clinical purposes, these questionnaires appear to be appropriate as a first screen to identify patients with excessive pain-related fear. We have used the TSK in clinical research (see Chapter 6) as a screening tool. This program of research was initiated using the original 17-item TSK, and data obtained from clinical populations gave mean scores on the questionnaire in the range between 38 and 40 (the range of possible scores is 17–68), and we have generally used a cut score of 39/40 to select patients for further detailed assessment of suitability for treatment. Norms for the newer 11-item version have been developed using a linear regression method that enables more precise interpretation of an individual's score that takes into account their gender and diagnosis [29]. Future research should enable the development of more precise selection criteria. At present, we recommend that individuals with scores above the mean be considered for further assessment.

Although questionnaires provide an initial profile of significant components of the fear-avoidance model, they do not give us specific information about the individual's fearful avoidance behavior, the context in which the behavior occurs, or information about more subtle safety-seeking behaviors that may be associated with avoidance. To assess these aspects further, we need to conduct a clinical interview.

Semi-Structured Interview

The semi-structured interview is an additional and important tool for obtaining information regarding the cognitive, behavioral, and psychophysiological aspects of the symptoms and to provide a better estimate of the role of pain-related fear in the maintenance of the pain problem. It also includes information regarding the antecedents (situational or internal) of the pain-related fear, the cognitive appraisals of pain, and the direct and indirect consequences of fear. The interview may also include other areas of life stresses because they might increase arousal levels and indirectly fuel pain-related fear.

During the interview, more specific information can be obtained on the patient's assumptions about the relationships between specific aspects of their physical activity, their pain experience, and their belief that (re)injury will occur. Beliefs of fearful patients with chronic pain often take the form of conditional assumptions of the type, "If P, then Q," where P is the predictor of a catastrophic consequence (Q). These predictions can be very specific and may contain detailed information about the patient's causal beliefs. For example, a patient might say something like, "If I lift a crate with bottles of soda from the ground with straight legs, then nerves become overexcited, which leads to permanent loss of control of the legs," or make a more general statement such as, "If I feel pain, it means that my injury is getting worse." Often these forms of reasoning follow a confirmation bias in the sense that the rule, "If P, then Q" is seldom falsified. To challenge and falsify the belief, we need to establish tests of instances in which P is followed by non-Q. In the case of dysfunctional assumptions, selectively searching for confirming evidence and the lack of falsifying evidence might reinforce the credibility of the false assumptions [31].

It has to be kept in mind that patients with chronic pain do not usually conceive of their problem as a phobia, and they may not talk about fear. As a consequence, the assessment interview should be sensitive to the probable discrepancy between the expert clinician's understanding of the problem and the patient's perception. Most patients are concerned with harm that may occur if they ignore the meaning of pain as they construe it, and we suggest that the interview be geared toward the patient's perception of their pain problem. Based on our experience, we would rather paraphrase their personal story in terms of harmfulness ("You feel that it might be better not to lift with straight legs" or, "I understand that you expect that this activity might further harm the nerves in your back") rather than using the words fear and anxiety, which themselves may be alarming. The role of pain-related fear is first evident during the educational part of the exposure treatment. We often observe that patients later during treatment spontaneously start reconceptualizing their pain problem as a problem of the overestimation of danger and excessive avoidance behavior.

Although many patients with chronic musculoskeletal pain have similar fears (fear of physical activities that produce pain or that are assumed to cause re-injury), the origin of their fears may be different. As discussed in Chapter 2, fears can be acquired along the following three pathways: direct experience, observational learning, and verbal instruction [26]. Each of these can be recognized in the pain histories of fearful patients who seek treatment. Making the origins of their fear clearer to the patient can be helpful when presenting the formulation and rationale for treatment (see Chapter 4). From clinical observation, we note that several factors that often appear to be associated with the development of fear are the characteristics of pain onset, particularly unpredicted traumatic events and ambiguity around the presence or absence of positive medico-diagnostic findings, and the information relayed to the patient by health care professionals. For example, an individual involved in a traffic accident might develop a fear of driving as a result of the traumatic experience. They might believe that movements necessitated by driving, for example, turning and twisting to check the whereabouts of traffic, might lead to further damage. Likewise, a patient with back pain might develop a fear of lifting after experiencing pain while lifting or after receiving information from a medical doctor that lifting can damage nerves in the spinal cord. We note that health care professionals might give rather complex messages that can be hedged with suitable cautions and caveats that are essentially accurate. However, patients might not hear or understand the subtlety of the message but simply extract the simplest and most threatening aspects of the message. Our clinical observations are that most patients with chronic back pain who present with pain-related fear appear to base their conviction about their vulnerability to (re)injury on results of diagnostic imaging (radiographic or magnetic resonance imaging [MRI]) tests. The combination of (threatening) information conveyed by the medical specialist and the experience of pain and discomfort appear to strengthen that conviction. The visual confrontation with radiographs or MRI images and simply hearing the diagnosis can be quite upsetting to some patients. This information might be interpreted as being more threatening than is intended by the specialist. Witnessing another person being severely disabled as a result of chronic pain might also be a source of information that strengthens the threat value of pain, even without actually experiencing these consequences. There is accumulating evidence that fear of pain can be acquired by observing others in pain [13]. Although we can rarely be absolutely sure about the etiological mechanisms in individual cases, reports about misconceptions and misinterpretations of information and the patient's experiences of others in pain can be useful. Collating the patient's experiences and integrating them into a formulation (case conceptualization) that is presented to the patient in the educational part of the intervention (Chapter 5) is an effective way of communicating the patient's framework.

The interview is also used to identify the current level of severity and maintaining factors of the pain problem and associated pain-related fear. The severity can often be estimated by inquiring about the extent to which the pain problem interferes with daily life, including the ability to carry out paid work, leisure activities, and normal relationships. Maintaining factors are usually negative thoughts about the danger of the physical activities, the avoidance of these activities, and hypervigilance to signals of threat. Negative thoughts can be elicited by inquiring about the patient's personal theory about his or her pain and associated functional incapacity. The experience of chronic pain generates profound fears for the individual's future that frequently include increased physical disability and social isolation [16,24]. If the patient believes that these fears are more likely to be realized if they fail to control the pain or prevent further injury, then they will be motivated to avoid what they believe to be threatening activities. Thus, expectations about the future, especially what they fear might happen, are investigated (e.g., "What do you think will happen if the pain is left untreated?"). For example, a female patient with back and pelvic pain, complaints that began during her first pregnancy and increased after delivery, started worrying about the future. Gentle questioning revealed that she had a relative who had received the same diagnosis and had finally become wheelchair bound. Her main belief was that during certain movements, the tissue and nerves around the ridged symphysis pubis could be damaged or ruptured, possibly resulting in paralysis of the lower limbs. In most cases, thoughts of probable harm alert individuals to bodily sensations that might signal impending danger. Situations that provoke these sensations are fearfully avoided. To gain insight into avoidance behaviors, the therapist may ask questions such as, "What does the pain prevent you from doing?" and, "If you no longer had this pain problem, what differences would it make to your daily life?" One can also ask directly about situations that might worsen the pain problem.

Finally, the assessment also includes clarifications about whether other problems, such as major depression, marital conflicts, or disability claims, warrant specific attention before or after treatment. In some cases, when more complicated problems are expected to arise if the pain problem were to diminish, it may also be warranted to leave the pain disability problem untreated. In practice, it is difficult to provide hard and fast rules about when one would decide *not* to offer treatment using graded in vivo exposure, and a degree of clinical judgment must enter into the equation. One common issue is the presence of ongoing legal compensation claims after trauma in which a third party is involved. Patients might understandably wish to maintain a level of disability to enhance the magnitude of compensation that they might attract. Their sense of justice and entitlement to sufficient compensation can conflict with the motivation to engage in treatment that would essentially remove evidence of their suffering. A second major consideration is the presence of depression, which is frequently comorbid with chronic pain [1]. For many individuals, depression is secondary to chronic pain, and the experience of depression in pain can be subtly different from depression in a mental health setting where chronic pain is not present. We suggest that a significant feature is the cognitive focus of negative thoughts. Whereas "normal" depression is often marked by a degree of self-denigration (self-hatred and loathing), patients with pain and depressed mood focus their negative thoughts on the pain rather than core aspects of the self [4,25]. The presence of depression does need careful consideration, and in many cases *active* treatment can be beneficial. Indeed, we note that a major effective treatment for depression in the mental health setting is behavioral activation; this approach is also based on the analysis of avoidance behavior [9]. Active treatment using the exposure protocol may therefore be an effective treatment in the presence of depression. Our major caveat is that working with seriously depressed patients does require appropriate risk assessments, and where necessary, liaison with a suitable mental health professional. Finally, exposure treatment might be difficult for patients who have pain reduction as their primary goal and who encounter difficulties in formulating functional goals independent of pain. Of course, the alleviation of pain is often the first goal that patients have in mind when they are asked, "What do you expect from this treatment?" Therefore, the very brief subsequent question, "What else?" might be a good way to elicit other goals as well, even if patients need some time and guidance to come up with other non–pain-related functional goals (such as playing with children again, working in the garden, resumption of job activities etc.). The inability to formulate such functional goals might be a third reason for not starting exposure treatment.

A summary of the topics covered during the interview is contained. The questions in Box 1 cover the main features of the fear-avoidance model. To illustrate this, we have mapped them onto the simple schematic representation of the model in Fig. 1. In many clinical

BOX 1
The Initial Screening Interview

Aim

To gather information on the cognitive, behavioral, and psychophysiological aspects of the pain complaints. To get a better understanding of the role of pain-related fear in the maintenance of the complaints and their interference with daily life activities.

Topics

1. Describe your current pain. (Affective quality, severity, location, course over the day)

2. What are the consequences of your pain problem for your daily life activities? (Work, household, leisure, social contacts, intimacy, family)

3. When did the pain start for the first time? (Experiential learning, traumatic event)

4. What is the course of your pain over time, from the start until now? (Changes, intermittent episodes, number of episodes, slowly increasing)

5. What are the things that can worsen or ease the pain? (Safety cues, eliciting cues)

6. Do you have control over the pain?

7. What do you do when the pain increases? (Escape, avoidance behavior, pacing)

8. What are you not doing anymore due to the pain? (Avoidance behavior)

9. How can other people see that you are in pain? (Pain behavior)

10. How do other people respond when they observe you in pain? (Social reinforcers)

11. What has changed in your life since you have been in pain? (Negative reinforcement)

12. What do you think is going on in your body? What do you think causes your pain? (Catastrophic interpretations)

13. Why do you think these are the causes of your pain? (Verbal and observational learning)

14. What is the cause of your pain as indicated by your physician? (Verbal learning)

15. What would happen if you were continue with your valued activities despite pain? (Threat value of pain)

16. What do you think will happen to your pain in the near future? (Expectancies)

17. What do you wish to attain with this treatment? (Goals)

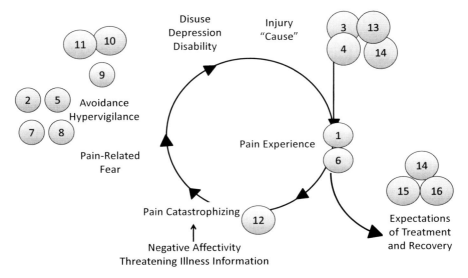

Fig. 1. This figure shows the relationship between the questions in Box 1 and a simple schematic representation of the fear-avoidance model.

interviews, it is not always possible to cover the questions in the order given in Box 1 because patients often need to tell their clinical story in their preferred manner. With practice, it is possible to retain the essential contents of the questions in Box 1 and to map the patient's answers onto the fear-avoidance model.

Developing Graded Hierarchies

Once we have established the applicability of the fear-avoidance model for a patient, we need to determine more precisely the essential stimuli that elicit the perception of threat and avoidance behaviors. Thus far, there are no standardized questionnaires for identifying these stimuli that are early in the chain of events leading to avoidance and protective safety behavior. Often, the stimuli are those that were immediately followed by the aversive event during the onset of pain, if such an onset can be recollected. In our experience, it is often difficult for patients with pain to estimate and report the threat value of different situations. One of the problems is that the avoidance behaviors are not really acknowledged as consequences of fear but as a direct consequence of the pain and the experienced vulnerability to (re)injury. In addition to checklists of daily activities, it is possible to use pictorial representations of movements that occur in everyday life, for example, lifting a shopping bag, getting into and out of a car, sweeping the yard, and using a vacuum cleaner, as prompts to elicit fear-related action. All of the activities just named are potentially back stressing and could elicit fear. In our experience, abrupt changes in movement (e.g., suddenly being hit) or activities consisting of repetitive spinal compressions (e.g., riding a bicycle on a bumpy road) are frequently mentioned stimuli by patients with chronic back and neck pain who score high on pain-related fear measures. These situations are feared because of idiosyncratic beliefs regarding the causes of pain such as ruptured or severely damaged nerves ("If I lift a crate with bottles of soda, the nerves in my back might be damaged"). Of interest is also that the same activity can be rated differently depending on the context in which the activity is performed. For example, the activity "running" can be considered quite harmful when performed in the woods and less harmful when performed on an even terrain.

We have developed several sets of photographs of daily activities that capture movement related to various parts of the body (back [19], neck [10], and upper and lower limbs [14]). They were designed to facilitate the development of graded hierarchies. The photographs cover the range of movements in all possible geometric plains and are capable of reflecting the full range of situations avoided by the patient, beginning with those that provoke only mild discomfort and ending with activities or situations that are beyond the patient's present abilities. The original measure, the Photograph Series of Daily Activities (PHODA) [17], is a standardized method that appears appropriate to design graded hierarchies. (An electronic version can be downloaded free of charge at http://www.psychology.unimaas.nl/phoda-sev). The PHODA uses 98 photographs representing various physical daily life activities including lifting, bending, walking, bicycling, etc. The photographs are presented to the patient, who is asked to place each photograph along a fear "thermometer." This scale consists of a vertical line with 11 anchor points (ranging from 0 to 100 in 10-point intervals) printed on 60 cm × 40 cm hardboard (Fig. 2). The fear thermometer is placed on a table in front of the patient with the following instructions: "Please look at each photograph carefully and try to imagine yourself performing the same movement. Place the photograph on the thermometer according to the extent to which you feel that this movement is harmful to your back." Note that we use the word "harmful" and that we do not ask the patient to directly rate their fear. The PHODA has shown good psychometric properties and has also been used to successfully measure not just harmfulness but also anticipated pain when performing imagined physical activities [34]. Further psychometric study using factor analysis has shown that it is possible to use a short electronic version (the PHODA-SeV), which measures a single factor and has a high internal consistency [19]. The test-retest reliability and stability of the PHODA-SeV over a 2-week period are good, and changes greater than 20 points between two occasions indicate a true change. The construct validity is supported by the finding that both self-reported pain severity and fear of movement/

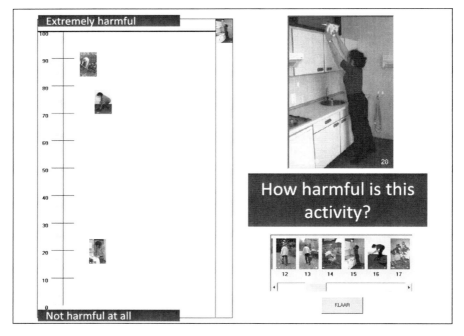

Fig. 2. A screen shot of the computerized version of the Photograph Series of Daily Activities (PHODA-SeV).

(re)injury are uniquely related to the PHODA-SeV. The PHODA has also been successfully applied to elderly individuals with pain [2]. Turk and colleagues in the US have developed a similar Pictorial Fear of Activity Scale-Cervical (PFActS-C) to assess fear in patients with cervical pain [35].

For both the PHODA and the PFActS-C, patients have to organize photographs of daily activities (PHODA) or movements (PFActS-C) in ascending order based on the extent to which they believe that performing these activities would be harmful. The resulting sorted set provides a personal hierarchy of fear-eliciting activities that can be used to guide exposure-based treatment.

Behavioral Tests

Sometimes, patients find it hard to really estimate the harmfulness of an activity when it has been avoided extensively. For cases in which even pictorial methods do not work, behavioral tests can be introduced. These consist of performing an activity that has been avoided previously while performance indices (such as time, distance, or number of repetitions) are measured. For example, during the assessment, during both the interview and administration of the PHODA, a patient indicated that he was not afraid of possible damage and that it was the pain that caused problems with performing certain activities. It is possible to check this statement with a brief behavioral test, as illustrated by the following exchange:

Therapist: "Could you lift this crate with bottles of soda for me?"
Patient: "You want me to lift this crate?"
Therapist: "Yes."
Patient: "Oh no, I won't do that!"
Therapist: "Why not?"
Patient: "Because it's bad for my back."
Therapist: "Bad for your back? What do you think would happen?"
Patient: "My nerves will get squeezed, and I'm afraid it may cause them to rupture, so that I'll no longer be able to walk."

Target behaviors can be derived from PHODA items, and in most cases the behavioral tests can be considered as a variant of the exercise tolerance test described by Fordyce [11]. To assess the extent to which avoidance occurs, patients are asked to perform the activity "until pain, weakness, fatigue or any other reason causes you to wish to stop" ([11] p. 170). Behavioral tests have the advantage that anticipatory anxiety and anxiety during exposure can be measured separately [3]. In addition, they provide a more objective measure of avoidance behavior.

Conclusion

The challenge of assessment is to identify patients for whom pain-related fear and the ensuing avoidance are a significant problem. A range of questionnaires have either been constructed or further developed. Alternative pictorial assessment methods have been developed for identifying movements and activities that are considered harmful, and automated activity monitoring devices have been utilized. An important aspect is the uncovering of propositional knowledge that patients have on the relationship between pain-eliciting, pain, and physical harm because the exposure sessions will be focused on systematically challenging these propositions. One particular difficulty is to objectively measure avoidance behavior. Reliable and valid assessment methods are still being developed, not just for avoidance of fear-eliciting activities but also for more subtle safety-seeking behaviors. Thorough assessment sets the stage for successful exposure treatment.

References

[1]   Banks SM, Kerns RD. Explaining high rates of depression in chronic pain: a diathesis-stress framework. Psychol Bull 1996;119:95–110.
[2]   Basler HD, Luckmann J, Wolf U, Quint S. Fear-avoidance beliefs, physical activity, and disability in elderly individuals with chronic low back pain and healthy controls. Clin J Pain 2008;24:604–10.
[3]   Butler G. Phobic disorders. In: Hawton K, Salkovskis PM, Kirk J, Clark DM, editors. Cognitive behaviour therapy for psychiatric problems: a practical guide. Oxford: Oxford University Press; 1989. p. 97–128.
[4]   Clyde Z, Williams AC. Depression and mood. In: Linton SJ, editor. New avenues for the prevention of chronic musculoskeletal pain and disability. Amsterdam: Elsevier; 2002. p. 105–21.
[5]   Crombez G, Bijttebier P, Eccleston C, Mascagni T, Mertens G, Goubert L, Verstraeten K. The child version of the pain catastrophizing scale (PCS-C): a preliminary validation. Pain 2003;104:639–46.
[6]   Crombez G, Vlaeyen JWS, Heuts PHTG, Lysens R. Pain-related fear is more disabling than pain itself: evidence on the role of pain-related fear in chronic back pain disability. Pain 1999;80:329–39.
[7]   DeGood DE, Shutty MS. Assessment of pain beliefs, coping and self-efficacy. In: Turk DC, Melzack R, editors. Handbook of pain assessment. New York: Guilford; 1992. p. 214–34.

[8]   DeGood DE, Tait RC. Assessment of pain beliefs and coping. In: Turk DC, Melzack R, editors. Handbook of pain assessment. New York: Guilford; 2001. p. 320–45.

[9]   Dimidjian S, Barrera M, Martell C, Muñoz RF, Lewinsohn PM. The origins and current status of behavioral activation treatments for depression. Ann Rev Clin Psychol 2011;7:1–38.

[10]   Dubbers AT, Vikström MH, J.R. DJ. The Photograph Series of Daily Activities (PHODA): cervical spine and shoulder. CD-Rom version 1.2. Maastricht: Hogeschool Zuyd, University Maastricht and Institute for Rehabilitation Research; 2003.

[11]   Fordyce WE. Behavioral methods for chronic pain and illness. St Louis: Mosby; 1976.

[12]   George SZ, Lentz TA, Zeppieri G, Lee D, Chmielewski TL. Analysis of shortened versions of the Tampa Scale for Kinesiophobia and Pain Catastrophizing Scale for patients after anterior cruciate ligament reconstruction. Clin J Pain 2012;28:73–80.

[13]   Goubert L, Vlaeyen JW, Crombez G, Craig KD. Learning about pain from others: an observational learning account. J Pain 2010;12:167–74.

[14]   Jelinek S, Germes D, Leyckes N, De Jong JR. The Photograph Series of Daily Activities (PHODA-LE): low extremities. CD-Rom version 1.2. Maastricht: Hogeschool Zuyd, University Maastricht and Institute for Rehabilitation Research; 2003.

[15]   Jensen MP, Karoly P. Pain-specific beliefs, perceived symptom severity, and adjustment to chronic pain. Clin J Pain 1992;8:123–130.

[16]   Kindermans HP, Goossens ME, Roelofs J, Huijnen IP, Verbunt JA, Morley S, Vlaeyen JW. A content analysis of ideal, ought, and feared selves in patients with chronic low back pain. Eur J Pain 2010;14:648–53.

[17]   Kugler K, Wijn J, Geilen M, de Jong J, Vlaeyen JWS. The photograph series of daily activities (PHODA). Heerlen, The Netherlands: Institute for Rehabilitation Research and School for Physiotherapy; 1999.

[18]   Larsen DK, Taylor S, Asmundson GJ. Exploratory factor analysis of the Pain Anxiety Symptoms Scale in patients with chronic pain complaints. Pain 1997;69:27–34.

[19]   Leeuw M, Goossens ME, van Breukelen GJ, Boersma K, Vlaeyen JW. Measuring perceived harmfulness of physical activities in patients with chronic low back pain: the Photograph Series of Daily Activities—short electronic version. J Pain 2007;8:840–9.

[20]   Lefebvre MF. Cognitive distortion and cognitive errors in depressed psychiatric and low back pain patients. J Consult Clin Psychol 1981;49:517–25.

[21]   McCracken LM, Dhingra L. A short version of the Pain Anxiety Symptoms Scale (PASS-20): preliminary development and validity. Pain Res Manage 2002;7:45–50.

[22]   McCracken LM, Zayfert C, Gross RT. The Pain Anxiety Symptoms Scale: development and validation of a scale to measure fear of pain. Pain 1992;50:67–73.

[23]   Miller RP, Kori SH, Todd DD. The Tampa Scale: a measure of kinesiophobia. Clin J Pain 1991;7:51–2.

[24]   Morley S, Eccleston C. The object of fear in pain. In: Asmundson GJ, Vlaeyen J, Crombez G, editors. Understanding and treating fear of pain. Oxford: Oxford University Press; 2004. p. 163–88.

[25]   Pincus T, Morley S. Cognitive processing bias in chronic pain: a review and integration. Psychol Bull 2001;127:599–617.

[26]   Rachman S. The conditioning theory of fear-acquisition: a critical examination. Behav Res Ther 1977;15:375–87.

[27]   Riley JF, Ahern DK, Follick MJ. Chronic pain and functional impairment: assessing beliefs about their relationship. Arch Phys Med Rehabil 1988;69:579–82.

[28]   Roelofs J, Goubert L, Peters ML, Vlaeyen J, Crombez G. The Tampa Scale for Kinesiophobia: further examination of psychometric properties in patients with chronic low back pain and fibromyalgia. Euro J Pain 2004;8:495–502.

[29]   Roelofs J, van Breukelen G, Sluiter J, Frings-Dresen MH, Goossens M, Thibault P, Boersma K, Vlaeyen JW. Norming of the Tampa Scale for Kinesiophobia across pain diagnoses and various countries. Pain 2011;152:1090–5.

[30]   Rosenstiel AK, Keefe FJ. The use of coping strategies in chronic low back pain. Pain 1983;17:33–44.

[31]   Smeets G, de Jong PJ, Mayer B. If you suffer from a headache, then you have a brain tumour: domain-specific reasoning 'bias' and hypochondriasis. Behav Res Ther 2000;38:763–76.

[32]   Sullivan MJL, Bishop SR, Pivik J. The Pain Catastrophizing Scale: development and validation. Psychol Assess 1995;7:524–32.

[33] Sullivan MJL, Thorn BE, Haythornthwaite JA, Keefe FJ, Martin M, Bradley LA, Lefebvre JC. Theoretical perspectives on the relationship between catastrophizing and pain. Clin J Pain 2001;17:52–64.

[34] Trost Z, France CR, Thomas JS. Examination of the photograph series of daily activities (PHODA) scale in chronic low back pain patients with high and low kinesiophobia. Pain 2009;141:276–82.

[35] Turk DC, Robinson JP, Sherman JJ, Burwinkle T, Swanson K. Assessing fear in patients with cervical pain: development and validation of the Pictorial Fear of Activity Scale-Cervical (PFActS-C). Pain 2008;139:55–62.

[36] Van Breukelen GJ, Vlaeyen JW. Norming clinical questionnaires with multiple regression: the Pain Cognition List. Psychol Assess 2005;17:336–44.

[37] Van Damme S, Crombez G, Bijttebier P, Goubert L, Van Houdenhove B. A confirmatory factor analysis of the Pain Catastrophizing Scale: invariant factor structure across clinical and non-clinical populations. Pain 2002;96:319–24.

[38] Vlaeyen J, van Breukelen G, Nooyen-Haazen IWCJ, Stomp-van den Berg SG, Kole-Snijders AM. Pijn cognitie lijst—2003. Maastricht: Academisch Ziekenhuis Maastricht, Pijn Kennis Centrum; 2003.

[39] Vlaeyen JW, Geurts SM, Kole-Snijders AM, Schuerman JA, Groenman NH, van Eek H. What do chronic pain patients think of their pain? Towards a pain cognition questionnaire. Br J Clin Psychol 1990;29:383–94.

[40] Vlaeyen JW, Kole-Snijders AM, Boeren RG, van Eek H. Fear of movement/(re)injury in chronic low back pain and its relation to behavioral performance. Pain 1995;62:363–72.

[41] Waddell G, Newton M, Henderson I, Somerville D, Main CJ. A fear-avoidance beliefs questionnaire (FABQ) and the role of fear-avoidance beliefs in chronic low-back-pain and disability. Pain 1993;52:157–68.

Essential Guide to Treatment

Although Wilbert Fordyce introduced the distinction between "hurt" and "harm" [19], Clare Philips was one of the first to argue for the systematic application of graded exposure to produce disconfirmations between expectations of harm and the actual consequences of painful activity [35]. She suggested, "These disconfirmations can be made more obvious to the sufferer by helping to clarify the expectations he or she is working with, and by delineating the conditions or stimuli which he feels are likely to fulfill his expectations. Repeated, graded, and controlled exposures to such situations under optimal conditions are likely to produce the largest and most powerful disconfirmations" ([35] p. 279). Experimental support for this idea is provided by the match-mismatch model of pain. This model conjectures that individuals initially tend to overpredict how much pain they will experience, but after some exposure, these predictions tend to be corrected to match with the actual experience [36]. Crombez and colleagues tested the model in patients with chronic low back pain [13]. The patients were to perform four exercise bouts (two with each leg) at maximal force. During each exercise bout, baseline pain, expected pain, and experienced pain were recorded. As predicted, the patients initially overpredicted pain, but after repetition of the exercise bout, the overprediction was readily corrected. The expectancy did not appear to generalize to the exercise episode with the other leg because a small increase in the expected level of pain re-emerged. This overprediction was immediately corrected after another performance. These findings were replicated with two other physical activities, bending forward and raising a straight leg [22]. In summary, it appears plausible that by analogy with the treatment of anxiety disorders, graded exposure to back-stressing movements may indeed be a successful treatment approach for patients with pain who report substantial fear of movement/(re)injury.

In our first study, we treated four consecutive patients with a high fear of movement/(re)injury (Tampa Scale for Kinesiophobia [TSK] score >40). The patients were randomly assigned to one of two sequences of intervention. In sequence A, patients received exposure treatment first, followed by graded exercise training. In sequence B, the treatment module order was reversed. Daily measures of pain-related cognition and fears were recorded with visual analog scales. Time series analyses revealed improvements during the in vivo exposure but not during the graded exercise. Further analysis of the pre-post treatment differences revealed that decreases in pain-related fear concurred with decreases in experienced pain disability, suggesting that it was the fear of pain that hampered the performance of daily activities [42]. In a subsequent study, patients carried an ambulatory activity monitor at home for 1 week after each treatment module. Results were similar to those of the previous study, but additionally decreased pain-related fear also concurred with an increase in physical activity in the home setting [43]. Subsequent controlled studies with larger numbers of subjects, different settings, and other pain problems (including neck pain, upper extremity pain, and complex regional pain syndrome [CRPS]) confirmed these results. In the remainder of this chapter, we will describe in more detail the specifics of the in vivo exposure treatment developed for patients who report increased levels of pain-related fear and avoidance behavior. Chapter 5 provides a discussion of pitfalls and problems that the therapist might encounter during an in vivo exposure session. A critical overview of the effectiveness of in vivo exposure treatment is provided in Chapters 6 through 8, and ideas on future directions will be offered in Chapter 9. Brief film clips and practical materials for patients and therapists are provided in the accompanying DVD.

Graded Activity, In Vivo Exposure, and Behavioral Experiments

In Vivo Exposure Versus Graded Activity

At first glance, in vivo exposure might appear quite similar to the more widely applied graded activity programs [20,28], in that it gradually increases activity levels despite pain. However, both conceptually and practically, these treatments are quite different (see Table I). First, graded activity is based on instrumental (operant) learning principles, and selected behaviors are shaped by positively reinforcing a predefined quota of activities (for more information on graded activity, see [19,38]). In vivo exposure, which stems from the behavior therapy tradition, is

Table I
Differences between graded activity, in vivo exposure, and behavioral experiments

	Graded Activity	In Vivo Exposure	Behavioral Experiments
Theoretical basis	Operant conditioning. Changing pain-rest contingencies to reduce disabling pain behaviors and increase healthy behaviors	Respondent conditioning. Extinction of conditioned fear responses via exposure to the conditioned stimulus (e.g., physical activity) in the absence of the unconditioned stimulus (e.g., increased pain, physical harm)	Challenging cognitive "errors"
Treatment goal	To increase function despite pain by increasing/shaping healthy behaviors	To increase function by reducing pain-related fear and avoidance behaviors	To increase function by changing beliefs and correcting cognitive errors
Treatment preparation	Establishment of activity tolerance levels and identification of discriminative stimuli eliciting pain behaviors	Establishment of a pain-relevant fear hierarchy	Cognitive analysis of the pain-related beliefs
Typical treatment techniques	Positive reinforcement of successive approximations to preset functional goals	Graded exposure to fear-eliciting painful activities	Hypothesis testing via manipulation of patients' own behavior

the clinical analog of extinction of conditioned fear [3]. When an individual is exposed to a conditioned stimulus (CS) that is no longer followed by the unconditioned stimulus (US), the conditioned fear response that was elicited by the CS extinguishes. Second, during graded activity, special attention is paid to the identification of positive reinforcers that are presented when the individual's quota is met, whereas with in vivo exposure the therapist pays special attention to the establishment of a specific hierarchy of pain-related fear stimuli relevant to that particular individual. During in vivo exposure, emotional responses are monitored, and the procedure continues until the distress level is significantly reduced. Third, graded activity programs usually include individual exercises according to functional capacity and observed individual physical work demands, whereas in vivo exposure includes activities that are selected based on the fear hierarchy and the idiosyncratic aspects of the fear stimuli. For example, if the patient fears the repetitive spinal compression produced by riding a bicycle on a bumpy road, graded exposure usually includes that specific activity, whereas graded activity more likely has the goal to ride a bike for a certain work load or duration.

In Vivo Exposure and Behavioral Experiments

There are similarities between exposure and behavioral experiments that are key treatment elements of cognitive therapy [1]. During behavioral experiments, patients are often exposed to situations that they have avoided for a long time, with the aim of challenging their belief that some behavior might worsen their condition. The validity of a certain target and alternative expectancies are closely monitored. Subsequent experiments are designed until the target proposition or belief is no longer considered valid. Despite conceptual differences, contemporary learning theory currently considers exposure not just an emotional, but also a cognitive process during which fear is activated and catastrophic expectations are challenged and disconfirmed. This results in a reduction of the threat value of the originally fearful stimulus. This is in line with the idea that inhibitory learning is at stake during exposure. Because the learned CS-US associations are not erased from memory, a competition occurs between the early CS-US and the novel CS-no US associations. Because in vivo exposure and behavioral experiments likely act on similar mechanisms, they can be combined. Common to all three approaches, the intervention is structured around the following four phases: education, defining treatment goals, establishing a fear hierarchy, and the actual exposure to feared stimuli. The exposure treatment that is described in the remaining of this chapter is based on the most up-to-date guidelines for the treatment of fear-related problems including those for cognitive-behavioral treatments [2,7] and for the application of behavioral interventions for chronic pain [39,41]. Before we discuss the elements of exposure in detail, we introduce two case examples, one of a patient with chronic back pain and one of a patient with CRPS, both of whom were referred for treatment because of their increased levels of pain-related fear and disability.

Two Case Illustrations

George

George was a 56-year-old married accountant with chronic back pain. He and his wife owned a farmhouse, and he had the intention of working less in order to keep and enjoy a small flock of sheep. For this purpose, he was working 60 to 70 hours a week in his home office. Four years earlier, he had witnessed a car crash on the street in front of his house. The car failed to take a bend and crashed into a tree. The driver was trapped in the car, and George tried to rescue him. When he pulled the victim out of the wreck, he suddenly heard a crack in his own back. He did not feel pain immediately, but when the emergency services arrived and he observed the situation at a certain distance, he felt a shooting pain is his back. The next day, the pain increased, and George decided to consult his general practitioner, who told him that the pain was probably caused by a muscle sprain and prescribed bed rest together with anti-inflammatory drug treatment. George's pain persisted, and subsequent treatments, including transcutaneous electrical nerve stimulation, physiotherapy, osteopathy, manual therapy, and wearing a corset, were unsuccessful. Finally George stopped working. A neurologist induced nerve blocks that relieved the pain for about 1 month, after which the pain returned. Finally, George was referred for treatment at a comprehensive rehabilitation program. The psychological assessment revealed that George was quite fearful. He was convinced that the vertebrae in his back had been damaged. He was concerned that any extra load on his back would worsen his pain condition and that there was a serious risk that he would end up in a wheelchair. George's core propositions were, "If I perform a lifting movement, my pain will increase" and more importantly, "If my pain worsens, the risk of damage to my spine increases." Given his main life goal to stop working as an administrator and start a small farm in the countryside, his more specific goals were focused on anticipated activities associated with farming, lifting and pulling weights in particular.

Lotte

Lotte, a 30-year-old woman, fell off her bike 5 years prior and fractured her right leg. Despite successful healing of the bone, her pain continued, and the skin of the lower leg gradually became red, warm, and swollen, with excessive hair growth, typical symptoms of CRPS type I. The associated allodynia prevented her standing and walking. She visited different physicians, and several treatments were initiated including pharmacotherapy, nerve blockade, transcutaneous electrical nerve stimulation, and physiotherapy. Despite these interventions, her pain complaints as well as the physiological signs/symptoms increased, and gradually the symptoms started to interfere with her daily life. Physical contact of the skin by any object became so painful that she stopped wearing shoes and fitted clothing. Because walking was only possible with the support of crutches, she disengaged fully from most of her usual daily activities. For example, Lotte became unable to play with her 3-year-old daughter in a natural and spontaneous manner. As a result of her incapacitation, she received workers' compensation. Lotte's understanding of her symptoms was that the pain and swelling of her leg was the result of overuse of muscles and nerves. She was absolutely convinced that connective tissue was damaged and that painful movement would result in further bodily damage that might ultimately lead to amputation of the leg (an option that she had read about in a magazine). Lotte's core propositions were, "If I am physically active, my pain will increase," and "If I do things that increase pain, the muscle tissue in my leg will decay."

Treatment Phase 1: Education and Preparing a Formulation

After the initial assessment, which may take one or two sessions, at least one session is devoted to providing information about the background and goals of treatment. Patients who are convinced that certain movements will harm their body usually are reluctant to engage in activities that challenge their basic assumptions about the "movement-pain-injury" sequence. Helping patients engage in exposure sessions therefore begins with an education phase during which the therapist presents an individualized formulation of the pain problem. The goal here is to help patients reframe their pain experience and to correct any misconceptions that have occurred early on during the development of the pain-related fear. Ideally, their experience is reframed as a common condition that can be self-managed, rather than as some serious disease that needs careful protection. The other major goal of the educational part is to increase the willingness of the patient to engage in valued activities that have been avoided for a long time. Preferably, an educational session is given by both the psychologist and a medical specialist. This combination of professionals generally increases the perceived credibility of the new information provided to the patient (see Guideline Boxes 1 and 2).

Guideline Box 1
Information provided by the medical specialist.

1. Prepare for the session by obtaining diagnostic materials, such as radiographs, magnetic resonance imaging (MRI) scans, and laboratory results.
2. Ask about the patient's medical history and discuss contradictions between earlier diagnoses and the current diagnosis.
3. Discuss the medical findings and make sure that the patient understands them. Avoid complex terminology.
4. Explain age-related abnormalities when present, and tell the patient that these findings are seen in symptom-free individuals as well.
5. Explain that back pain is seldom caused by serious pathologies.
6. Assure that there are no medical reasons for not doing normal daily activities and that on the contrary, activity is necessary for maintaining a healthy body.
7. Explain that the absence of a serious pathology by no means indicates a psychological disorder.

Guideline Box 2
Providing an alternative rationale.

1. Prepare for the session by obtaining a flip-chart or whiteboard.

2. Ask about the latest meeting with the medical specialist, and check whether the patient has understood the information of the present medical status.

3. Indicate that the absence of serious pathology, despite severe pain, does not mean that pain is purely "in the mind" or "imagined" and that the pain is taken seriously by all staff.

4. Tell the patient that you think that he/she is capable of doing much more than he/she is doing now, probably with less pain.

5. Using interactive information, fill in specifics of the graphical representation of the fear-avoidance model (e.g., Figs. 3 and 4) with the idiosyncratic features of the patient's pain problem.

6. Give the patient ample opportunity to fill in the figure with his or her own words and terminology. Although all elements of the model are equally important, pain as a central problem is often a good starting point.

7. Discuss that in most cases, the real cause is unknown, but there are some other aspects that are relevant such as pain-related thoughts and beliefs, feelings and emotional responses, avoidance behavior, and long-term consequences.

Dialog Box 1 presents a typical example of a dialog based on Lotte, who met the psychologist after having received information from the medical specialist. The educational part is much more than just reassuring the patient that there are no specific physical abnormalities. In the absence of an alternative explanation for the pain problem and the associated functional limitations, mere reassurance that there is nothing wrong can have paradoxical and opposite effects [8,29,31]. To help counter this, the patient is given a careful explanation of the fear-avoidance model, using the patient's individual symptoms, beliefs, and behaviors to illustrate a how vicious cycle (pain → catastrophic thought → fear → avoidance → disability → pain) maintains the pain problem. Figs. 1 and 2 show the specific diagrammatic representations of formulations for George and Lotte based on the generalized schema of Fig. 3 of Chapter 1.

In cases where the pain-related fear appears to be related to the patient's previous experiences with diagnostic tests (radiography, magnetic resonance imaging [MRI]), it may be useful to review these tests together

---

Dialog Box 1
(TH = Therapist, PA = Patient)

TH: You just talked to the physician about the medical tests that were carried out a week ago. Can you tell me more about that?

PA: Well, we both looked at the scans, and they appeared less alarming than I thought. Apparently there are no fractures, and no trapped nerves. The doctor said that the scans show some wear and tear, but that this is not unusual for a person of my age.

TH: How was it for you to hear this information?

PA: Well, some relief because there is nothing dangerous going on. At the same time, difficult to understand … because why is it that I have so much pain and cannot walk or lift properly? There must be some reason.

TH: In people suffering from chronic pain such as yourself, it is not unusual to see that the medical diagnostics are quite normal and that there are no signs of physical damage.

PA: Are you suggesting that my pain is all imagined?

---

with a medical specialist. The purpose of this consultation is to explain to the patient that they have probably overestimated the value of these tests and that in symptom-free individuals, similar abnormalities can also be found. In this context, informing patients about study findings that reveal

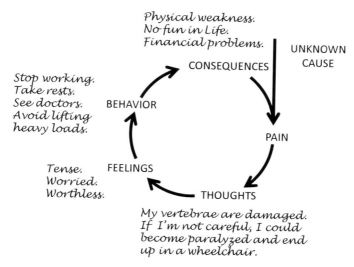

Fig. 1. Diagrammatic formulation for George.

that individuals with and without back pain have similar MRI scans suggests that the relevance of these imaging techniques in individuals with chronic pain is rather limited [24]. In addition, the therapist can advise the patient to read one of the existing patient-centered books or leaflets such as the British "Back Book" [5,6,21,26].

Education is the first step toward enhancing the commitment of the patient to engage in feared activities during the actual in vivo exposure. In the context of education, there is one field of research that has focused on *preventing* chronicity of low back pain by giving adequate *written* information. Burton and colleagues studied the effect of an educational booklet on the beliefs and functional outcomes of patients seeking primary care for an acute or recurrent episode of low back pain [6]. Patients receiving this biopsychosocially oriented booklet showed significantly more positive beliefs regarding activities and consequences of low back pain, as compared to those receiving a traditional booklet designed for patients seeking treatment in primary care for acute or recurrent low back pain. This positive effect was maintained over a 1-year follow-up period, and this group also showed a tendency to become less disabled than the group who received information that was biomedically oriented [6]. In another study, the experimental group was

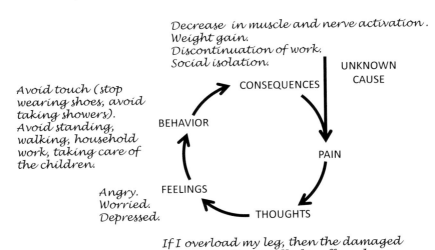

Fig. 2. Diagrammatic formulation for Lotte.

enrolled in a self-care program. This program consisted of two group sessions and an individual meeting with the psychologist leading the program, in which a plan was made to enhance self-care and problem-solving related to back pain. One follow-up telephone call was made to evaluate the patient's progress with this plan. Additional information was given by videos and a book; both emphasized the importance of resuming daily life activities. Control subjects only received a book about usual back pain care. The experimental intervention was effective in decreasing worries, pain intensity, and interference with activities. That is, repeated verbal information led to decreased pain-related fear in the experimental group, and to a lesser extent, reduced pain intensity and daily life interference, although a substantial number of patients continued to have back problems at the 6-month follow-up [32]. Note, however, that the patients included in both of these studies were not selected on the basis of their levels of pain-related fear. In a study of fearful patients [16], more fully reported in Chapter 7, we showed that a single educational session reduced self-reported fear of pain and pain catastrophizing, but that these ratings further diminished after the initiation of subsequent in vivo exposure. On its own, education was not powerful enough to change actual behavior; the performance of relevant daily activities was not affected by the educational session and improved significantly only with in vivo exposure. Education is a useful treatment component but not always sufficient to inhibit avoidance and more subtle safety behaviors.

One of the key elements of the educational session for patients with pain-related fear is to provide an *alternative explanation* for the symptoms, which is credible and integrates the idiosyncrasies of the patient's pain problem. The general point of the explanation is that the patient's safety behaviors are a normal defensive response to pain, which may have been adaptive in acute pain but have lost their efficacy as the pain has persisted. Over time, the defensive avoidance behavior will interfere with the performance of valued activities of daily life, which in turn might increase distress and aggravate the pain. The educational session is not meant to convince patients of the alternative explanation but to help them prepare for treatment and to increase their willingness to engage in the exposure sessions. In our experience, education works best when a medical specialist, who can explain that medical findings are absent or at least not indicative of serious pathology that requires prolonged caution (such as medication, supportive devices), is part of the treatment team. Sometimes, patients who have already consulted many specialists are quite skeptical about the possible outcome of any new treatment proposed (see Dialog Boxes 2 and 3).

The graphical presentation of the fear-avoidance model is a usual way to help patients understand that their own defensive behavior paradoxically may worsen the problem. In an interactive way (Dialog Box 4), the therapist tries to map out beliefs, feelings, behaviors, and their consequences. If the patient accepts that there may be alternatives to a biomedical explanation of their pain problem, the educational session usually is a springboard to the first exposure session. When sufficient information regarding the thoughts, feelings, and behaviors during increased pain are gathered, the downward spiral in the graph can be completed (see Figs. 1 and 2 for the graphs used for George and Lotte).

At this point, the patient might understand that protective behaviors can serve a short-term goal (ease pain and reduce fear) but compromise long-term goals such as the resumption of valued life activities

---

Dialog Box 2
(TH = Therapist, PA = Patient)

TH: The physician told you that there is nothing medically wrong with your back and that, in principle, you may do whatever you wish. This sounds like a positive message, perhaps sufficient to resolve the limitations in your daily life that you experience. Have you been more active since the meeting with the physician?

PA: Of course not, because my pain has not diminished.

TH: Right. The pain is an obstacle for you to do the things that you want to do, even though you have been reassured that your back is not damaged. Let's have a closer look at your pain problem. It is very common for people with chronic pain to adapt and adjust their behavior, as a natural way to protect the body against further pain. Sometimes, however, this protective behavior may go astray and become counterproductive. We believe that this may be the case in your situation. Given what we know about your condition, we believe that you will be capable of doing significantly more than you are doing right now and that you are suffering more than needed.

Dialog Box 3
(TH = Therapist, PA = Patient)

PA: I have seen a lot of doctors, and so far none of them have been able to help me. Nobody could take away my pain.

TH: I understand, and this must be quite frustrating. How about taking another perspective and looking at other ways of improving your current life situation?

PA: What do you mean?

TH: Well, we think there may be a way of becoming more active by not trying to reduce pain first, but by analyzing what your activity pattern is first. Suppose you could be more active with the same level of pain, would that be an improvement?

PA: I suppose so.

---

and social roles. When the patient is ready to accept this, the next question is how to interrupt this cycle. The therapist might introduce the essence of the behavioral experiments, explaining that a powerful way to challenge the "activity-pain-injury" assumption is to stop avoiding and to test each of the assumptions against an alternative one that can be formulated as the "activity-pain-no injury" assumption (see Guideline Boxes 1 and 2 for practical guidelines for the educational session). A particular technique that can help increase the motivation of a patient to engage in exposure treatment is "motivational interviewing" [25]. The essential idea is that the clinician will be most effective when they adjust their intervention to correspond with the motivational stage of the patient. When a patient is not even considering treatment, the clinician might start raising doubts about the patient's current course of action by increasing the patient's perception of the risks and problems associated with the current (avoidance) behavior. If the patient has shown interest but is still hesitating, the clinician might tip the balance by strengthening the patient's perceived ability to make it through treatment. If patients has already made preparations to engage in treatment, the clinician's task is to help them determine the best course of action at this point. In addition to these specific strategies, the motivational interviewing approach emphasizes empathetic listening, frequent patient affirmations, and gentle persuasion.

Dialog Box 4
(TH = Therapist, PA = Patient)

TH:	Let's try to draw your own way of protecting against pain on the white board (use wizard displayed in Fig. 1). To start with, what have you learned to do so far when in pain?
PA:	Well, when my pain is really bad, I should keep still because otherwise a nerve may rupture.
TH:	I understand, so pain tells you something is wrong, and that you need to be still. You mentioned earlier that a week ago, while cleaning the house you experienced a sudden pain increase, right? How did you feel?
PA:	I felt helpless, I couldn't move anymore, and I was scared that I was going to become paralyzed.
TH:	I can imagine that if you think that pain signals bodily damage and that when cleaning increases your back pain, then you become quite concerned. What did you do after feeling scared?
PA:	I stopped cleaning and lay down for a while.
TH:	Did the pain go away?
PA:	Not really. It went down a bit, but it came back later. The pain did not go away.
TH:	May I conclude that the "solution" of stopping activities when pain increases is not working well?
PA:	Well, it helps for a while, but it does not solve the problem.
TH:	The advantage of taking rests is that it eases the pain for a while. Are there also disadvantages of stopping activities?
PA:	I don't know … but I do not feel happy with doing so little.
TH:	Yes, it is quite possible that not doing activities that are important to you can be frustrating and may get you down.
PA:	I used to be an active person, working for my family. Now I feel worthless.
TH:	There also might be physical effects as well. What do you think are the effects of inactivity on your physical condition?
PA:	It hasn't got any better … I've also gained weight.

Treatment Phase 2: Determining Treatment Goals

After provision of an alternative framework aimed at helping the patient better understand how beliefs, feelings, and behaviors might maintain the chronic pain problem, there are several reasons why it is wise to also spend some time determining treatment goals [27]. First, cognitive-behavioral treatments for pain, including in vivo exposure, never aim at the reduction of pain but at the restoration of functional abilities despite pain. It helps to make this general goal explicit, and both patient and therapist should agree on one or more realistic and specific goals that are formulated in positive terms. If reduction of pain is the only or the most important goal, then exposure treatment might not be the right choice. Typical examples of suitable treatment goals are lifting a child, lifting a shopping bag, using a bicycle, walking to the supermarket alone, or resuming swimming. More general life goals, such as returning to work, taking up household chores, or going on holiday, can best be broken down into subgoals or smaller activities that can each be a subject for an in vivo exposure session. Goals are best formulated according to popular SMART guidelines, for which the acronym refers to goals being specific, measurable, attainable, rewarding, and time-bound [4]. The key question always remains why does the patient consider such a life goal not achievable at the moment? There might be specific movements involved that the patient is convinced are harmful, or there might be other obstacles leading to additional behavioral experiments. Second, setting goals also helps to structure the treatment and to design the hierarchy of stimuli that will be introduced during the actual in vivo exposure sessions. For example, if a patient wishes to resume sports activities, the therapist will make sure that aspects of these will be included in the graded exposure activities. Third, setting functional goals also redirects the focus of attention from pain and physical symptoms toward daily life activities with the emphasis on the possibility of change away from disability status. Finally, as the patient is invited to formulate his or her own goals, goal-setting inadvertently reinforces the notion that active participation is an essential part of treatment. Guideline Box 3 gives some practical guidelines for the session on establishing treatment goals.

Treatment Phase 3: Establishing a Fear Hierarchy

The goal of this session is not only to identify activities that the patient is avoiding but also to decide which activities will be selected for subsequent exposure sessions. By means of the Photograph Series of Daily Activities (PHODA; see Chapter 3), patients can sort photographs of various daily life

---

Guideline Box 3
Defining treatment goals.

---

1. There are a number of questions that can be used to help patients define their
   treatment goals:
   a. Why are you seeking help at our center?
   b. What would you be doing if you didn't have pain?
   c. What is the minimal change that would be satisfying for you?
   d. How would life be better for you?
2. If the patient mentions pain reduction or pain relief as the primary goal,
   acknowledge this and ask for other treatment goals, for example, "I understand
   that you would like to get rid of the pain, but what else would you like to occur?"
3. Sometimes patients come up with treatment goals during assessment of the fear
   hierarchy, when they are exposed to pictures of various daily activities, many of
   which they are not doing anymore because of the pain problem.

---

activities on a "harm thermometer" ranging from 0 (this is not harmful at
all) to 100 (this is extremely harmful). Note that patients are explicitly asked
not to judge photographs on the degree of anticipated painfulness but on
the expected *harmfulness* of the activity. This is important because painfulness is more difficult to challenge during the exposure sessions, whereas for
most patients, there is an overestimation of harm, which can be challenged.
Given that the PHODA includes a standardized set of daily activities, the
therapist will always include a blank photograph with the question, "Can
you think of any activity that is important to you, that you have not seen
so far, and which you think may be harmful to your body?" The patient's
response to the question is written on the blank photograph, which the patient subsequently can place on the thermometer. If necessary, more than
one blank photograph can be added to the series to ensure that the idiosyncratic aspects of the patients fear system are fully recognized. Table II
presents the fear hierarchies established for George and Lotte.

Treatment Phase 4:
Graded In Vivo Exposure
With Behavioral Experiments

Current treatments for excessive fears and anxiety are based on Wolpe's
work on systematic desensitization [45]. The essence of this treatment

method is that individuals progress through increasingly more anxiety-provoking encounters with phobic stimuli while using relaxation to inhibit their rising anxiety. Because relaxation was intended to compete with the anxiety response, a graded format was chosen to keep the anxiety level as weak as possible. However, later studies revealed that the *exposure* to the feared stimuli appeared to be most essential component of systematic desensitization and that it could be applied without relaxation to produce comparable effects [10]. For fearful patients, first-hand experience of behaving differently is far more convincing than rational argument. The essential step consists of graded exposure to the situation the patient has identified as "dangerous" or "threatening." Subsequently, individually tailored practice

Table II
Fear hierarchy for George and Lotte

Harm rating	George	Lotte
100	Pick up a crate of bottles Push a wheelbarrow Dig in the garden Play badminton	Cycle Jump
95		Run
90	Mow the lawn Paint Run downstairs	Climb stairs
80		Walk without crutches
75		
70	Rake Do fitness training Go mountain-biking Bend forward	Pick up a child
60		Stand (for a long time)
50	Swim Walk on dirt roads Squat Perform a twisting motion Sit on the couch Push the garbage container	Cut nails Touch
40		Wear socks
30	Turn over in bed Tie shoelaces	Cross legs

tasks are developed based on the graded hierarchy of fear-eliciting situations, and the general principles for exposure are followed, in which the patient agrees to perform certain activities or movements that they used to avoid. Each activity or movement is first modeled by the therapist, thereby demonstrating that it is a safe thing to do. The presence of the therapist, who may serve as an initial safety signal to promote more exposure, is gradually withdrawn to facilitate independence and to create a context that mimics that outside of treatment. The patient is encouraged to engage in these fearful activities as much as possible until disconfirmation has occurred and anxiety levels have decreased. This can be monitored by asking the patient to report subjective units of distress on a scale from 0 to 10 and to repeat the exposure task until the level of distress has decreased substantially. Another possibility is to ask the patient to move the PHODA items on the perceived harmfulness scale because some patients might generalize extinction of fear for one activity to similar activities, even though research has shown that generalization of extinction is quite slow [12,40].

As mentioned earlier, in vivo exposure often takes the form of a behavioral experiment. Guideline Boxes 4, 5, and 6 give details for the planning, execution, and evaluation of exposure-based behavioral experiments.

Guideline Box 4
Preparation for exposure to behavioral experiments.

1. Discuss homework (if appropriate).
2. Make sure that the purpose of the experiment is clear to the patient.
3. Select an activity with an appropriate level of difficulty, according to the fear hierarchy. Aiming too high or too low can be demoralizing and discouraging to the patient.
4. Specify the target expectancy and predicted outcome (if …, then …).
5. Specify the alternative expectancy and alternative outcome (if …, then …).
6. Have the patient rate the credibility of both expectancies (0–100%).
7. Decide what resources (place, time, materials, people) are needed.
8. Prepare the patient by stating that pain might increase during the experiment, but that this is a normal response.
9. Is the patient confident enough to embark on the exposure/experiment?
10. Do you feel confident in carrying out the exposure/experiment with this patient?
11. Anticipate possible problems, and work out measures to overcome them.

It is often mistakenly believed that cognitive therapy assumes that cognitive "errors" can be corrected simply via conscious reasoning, and behavioral experiments are an essential part of therapy. The essence of a behavioral experiment is that the patient performs an activity to challenge the validity of their catastrophic assumptions and misinterpretations. These assumptions take the form of, "If P, then Q" statements and are empirically tested during a behavioral experiment. Three steps can be distinguished. First, the patient formulates a hypothesis with the guidance of the therapist. For example, "If I jump down off a stair, then I will inevitably experience nerve damage in the spine and excruciating pain." Second, a one-session experiment is designed. For example, if the patient is convinced that jumping down is harmful, the therapist can further inquire about the minimal height that the patient considers necessary to cause nerve injury. Finally, the experiment is carried out and evaluated. After having modeled the activity, the therapist invites the patient to jump down off the stair, and the experienced consequences are evaluated. In practice, behavioral experiments are difficult to separate from mere exposure, and they can best be used simultaneously. Thus, in addition to monitoring changes in distress, as in exposure, the evaluation of each behavioral experiment determines changes in the beliefs that the patient holds regarding particular activities. For example, these can be monitored by asking patients to predict the occurrence of harm before the experiment and repeating the same question after exposure to that activity, "How would you rate the probability (0–100) that you will be unable to move after doing this activity?" When the rating has decreased substantially, the therapist may consider moving on to the next item in the hierarchy.

Examples of Treatment: Lotte and George

Given Lotte's predictions, the therapist decided that it would be best to start with behavioral experiments that provided evidence that touching the skin would not necessarily lead to long-term worsening of the symptoms. Therefore, the first session consisted of rubbing the skin, gently and then a bit more vigorously, first with a soft cloth and later with a rough surface. In subsequent behavioral experiments, everyday activities, such as cutting fingernails, taking a shower and drying off with a towel, and wearing socks and shoes, tested the alternative prediction that these

Guideline Box 5
Actions during exposure to the behavioral experiment.

A behavioral experiment can be used in addition to an exposure test to enhance the effect of in vivo exposure. In essence, a behavioral experiment involves an activity that allows testing of the validity of catastrophic misinterpretations of the pain. The patient is encouraged to identify catastrophic thoughts and to consider alternative thoughts. Conducting the experiment allows for examination of the validity of both the catastrophic and alternative thoughts.

1. Select activity:
   Together with the patient, select an activity from the list of activities. Consider the structure of the list to determine at which level of fear to start. Start at a level that is neither too high nor too low. Ensure that the activity is practicable.

2. Agree on execution:
   Make clear agreements on the activity by asking the patient what it takes to convince them that they are right or wrong. Be as specific as possible about the activity. For example, how often and how far they should bend over, how much weight is to be lifted, how long the activity will take, etc.

3. Be specific about the catastrophic thought:
   Make the catastrophic thought concrete by asking the patient what he/she expects will happen (severe acute pain, injury). Go for answers like "If I do this, then ...". If the patient expects a particular activity to induce severe acute pain, make sure you do not test this expectation, because it may prove valid. What is relevant here is the expected consequence of acute pain in terms of injury or damage (e.g., "If I do this, I will suffer back injury" or, "If I lift this weight, I will not be able to stand up again" or, "If this is causing severe acute pain, I will be paralyzed").

4. Ask how strongly the patient believes the catastrophic thought:
   Ask the patient to indicate how convinced he/she is of the truth of the catastrophic thought.

5. Be specific about the alternative thought.

6. Model the activity:
   Activities are best modeled because of at least two reasons:
   a. By modeling the activity, the therapist implicitly shows that it is a common activity that other people can do without concern.
   b. Modeling the activity might prevent the patient from engaging in safety behaviors.

7. Invite the patient to perform the activity:
   Encourage the patient to continue carrying out the activity until the fear has sufficiently diminished and/or the validity of the catastrophic thought has been tested.

Guideline Box 5 (continued)
Actions during exposure to the behavioral experiment.

8. Evaluate the patient's thoughts on the experiment:
   a. Postexperiment credibility of catastrophic thought: ask the patient to indicate how credible he/she thinks the catastrophic thought is after the activity.
   b. Decreased credibility of catastrophic thought: the decrease in credibility of the catastrophic thought is the difference between the degree of credibility before and after the activity.
   c. Postexperiment credibility of alternative thought: ask the patient to indicate how credible he/she thinks the alternative thought is after the activity.
   d. Increased credibility of alternative thought: the increase in credibility of the alternative thought is the difference between the degree of credibility before and after the activity.
   e. Evaluation of behavioral experiment: evaluate the patient's thoughts on the activity.

---

activities might cause a temporary increase in symptoms but that these would wane within a couple minutes. After successful exposures to skin touching, movements with the affected leg were tested by swinging the leg and sitting with legs crossed. Thereafter, standing on both legs with and without crutches, and later in combination with daily activities, such as washing dishes, ironing, and taking care for the children, was added. In the later phases of treatment, exposure-based behavioral experiments were extended to walking with and without crutches and to include several daily life activities involving walking, walking on unpaved roads, and using different types of footwear. The final exposure sessions concerned speed-walking, running, jumping, and playing sports [15].

Guideline Box 6
Reflections after exposure to the behavioral experiment

1. How can the outcome of the experiment contribute to reduced pain-related fear and increased functioning in daily life?
2. Decide how progress can be carried forward via new experiences.
3. Design the next behavioral experiment.
4. Provide homework by asking the patient to repeat the activities in the home situation.

Dialog Box 2

Dialog between George and his therapist during a behavioral experiment
(TH = Therapist, G = George)

TH: OK, today we'll start with the next activity. Why don't we try lifting this empty crate. What do you think?

G: [Sighs] I don't think I can manage that.

TH: What do you think might happen?

G: I'm sure I'll get more pain. The disks in my back can't take such pressure. It may further damage the nerves there.

TH: How would you notice this?

G: My back will collapse, I won't be able to stand, and I may become paralyzed.

TH: How likely is it that this will happen when lifting this crate, on a scale of 0 (not likely) to 100 (very likely)?

G: I am not sure: around 70.

TH: OK, well why don't we try it and see what happens. I'll do it first, and then it's your turn.

At this point the therapist models the lifting task and invites George to do the same, and while George is holding the crate, the therapist continues to inquire about what is happening.

TH: Good. You're doing very well. How did it go?

G: OK, I guess. It did hurt somewhat, but my back could hold it quite well. It didn't collapse.

TH: Right, despite the pain, you managed to lift this crate, right? Suppose we do this again, how would you rate the chances of your becoming paralyzed?

G: Well, I would say a 40, but there wasn't a crack.

TH: Would the situation be different if you had felt a crack?

G: Oh yes, definitely.

TH: How could we induce such a crack?

G: When I was still working, I usually carried heavier weights than the one I just lifted.

TH: Shall we make this one a bit heavier?

G: [Laughs nervously] OK then.

George's biggest fear was that his dream of enjoying and working on the farm was no longer possible. He was 100% convinced that planned activities such as taking care of the meadows, trees, and animals, and the refurbishment of the farm would cause further damage to his back and that he might end up in a wheelchair. George and his wife had also looked forward to having more time for long walks. However, George had the idea that during walking the load on his vertebrae was too great. George saw walking as a basic condition to function in daily life. During the first three exposure sessions, George was exposed to all kinds of conditions related to walking, for example, walking on flat terrain or gravel, over arable land, up and down a hill, walking fast, and walking longer than 2 hours. On the fourth exposure session, George was challenged to run. When convinced that walking and running did not harm his back, George wanted to challenge himself by lifting. George was convinced that lifting, and in particular lifting products greater than 10 kg, would damage the vertebrae of the spine, thereby pinching nerves so that he would not be able to walk anymore. George was concerned about the possible effects of shock-loading and sudden movements on his back. First, he was exposed to lifting small

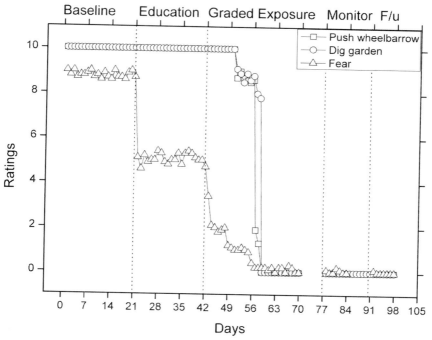

Fig. 3. Results of the exposure treatment for George. Baseline, followed by a 21-day no-treatment period; then a single education session, followed by a 21-day no-treatment period; followed by graded in vivo exposure. After this, George carried an ambulatory monitor (see Chapter 7) for 7 days, and 6 months later, he was followed up for 7 days.

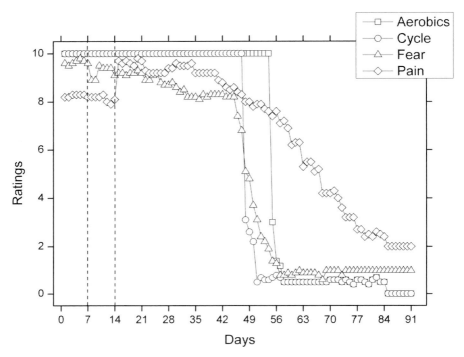

Fig. 4. Results of the exposure treatment for Lotte. The sequence of treatment phases was the same as for George in Fig. 3.

logs, followed by paint cans, tools, stepladders, a crate full of beer bottles, tiles, and finally straw bales that weighed about 20 to 25 kg (see Dialogue Box 5). In particular, the combination of bending forward and lifting was very threatening to George. Therefore, lift tasks were combined with walking, reaching, turning, throwing bales, and climbing the stairs. The last two exposure sessions, which he performed independently at home, were nonstop digging of a hole for a pond and using a tractor to plow arable land.

The results of exposure treatment for George and Lotte are displayed in Figs. 3 and 4, which show that the self-reported level of fear diminished after the educational session and diminished even more after the start of exposure. George was able to reach his two main goals (digging in the garden and pushing a wheelbarrow) after about 12 days of treatment. Lotte's treatment took a bit longer, but she was finally able to use her bicycle again and to join an aerobics club after 5 weeks of treatment. Also of interest is that Lotte was able to resume these valued activities before her pain levels reduced. At the end of the exposure treatment, pain intensity levels were reduced to an acceptable level.

Other Forms of Exposure

The in vivo form of graded exposure described earlier was developed specifically for patients with chronic musculoskeletal pain, and back pain in particular, who are severely disabled and who report substantial pain-related fear. Nevertheless, one has to bear in mind that there are several variations in the way exposure treatment can be conducted, most of which have not been systematically evaluated. One could for example consider *imagined* exposure [34] or exposure using *virtual reality* [33]. For patients with an ability to create vivid images, they may be asked to imagine that they are performing the "harmful" physical activities they tend to avoid. Instead of the consistent version we described (once every day for several weeks), a spaced form (once every week for several months) might also be an option. Rather than approaching the fearful stimuli in a graded fashion, an interesting question would be to what extent the process of change would be accelerated by directly exposing patients to the most intensely feared stimuli [9]. Thus far, this has not been tested, and of course, an obvious condition would be the willingness of the patients to engage in such an activity. In addition to exposure to painful movements, *interoceptive* exposure has been developed, in which the conditioned stimulus is considered to be within the body. Interoceptive exposure has been applied for patients with posttraumatic stress disorder [44], and the first results for patients with chronic pain are encouraging [11,17,18]. Finally, treatment would be made accessible to larger groups of patients if self-guided exposure with a manual is determined to be as effective as the therapist-guided exposure described here. The reason we have chosen graded exposure with the aid of a therapist is that based on our experience, we felt that it would provide the most credible, safe, and effective treatment approach. The final chapter will go into more detail regarding future developments in fear-reduction techniques in chronic pain.

Final Note: The Role of the Therapist

As mentioned, graded in vivo exposure might appear quite similar to the usual graded activity programs in that it gradually increases activity levels despite pain, but they are quite different, conceptually and as well as practically. As mentioned, in vivo exposure deals more directly with patients' emotions and cognitions than graded activity. This means that this type of treatment requires specific competencies in a therapist. Because in vivo exposure with behavioral experiments is a cognitive-behavioral intervention, training in cognitive-behavioral principles is a necessary prerequisite, and supervision by a psychologist experienced in the field of behavioral medicine, and the area of chronic pain in particular, is a sine qua non. In addition, the treatment will work best when delivered by therapists who are comfortable in exposing patients to movements and who are not fearful themselves that too much physical activity might harm the patient's physical condition. Rainville and colleagues conjectured that, "Patients' attitudes and beliefs (and thereby patients' disability levels) may be derived from the projected attitudes and beliefs of health care providers"([37] p. 288). A recent review concluded that there is moderate evidence that health care providers with a biomedical orientation (as compared to a behavioral orientation) or elevated fears of pain are more likely to advise patients to limit work and physical activities and are less likely to adhere to treatment guidelines [14,23]. It is expected that one's own fears will affect one's communication with patients and that one will experience more difficulty reassuring patients about the harmlessness of exposure sessions [30]. Regular training with and close supervision by an experienced cognitive-behavioral therapist who is working in the pain field might be a good start to gain sufficient confidence and skill in helping patients with chronic pain who report increased pain-related fear.

References

[1]   Beck A, Rush AJ, Shaw BP, Emery G. Cognitive therapy of depression. New York: Guilford Press; 1979.
[2]   Bennet-Levy J, Butler G, Fennell M, Hackman A, Mueller M, Westbrook D. Oxford guide to behavioural experiments in cognitive therapy. Oxford: Oxford University Press; 2004.
[3]   Bouton ME. Context and ambiguity in the extinction of emotional learning: Implications for exposure therapy. Behav Res Ther 1988;26:137–49.

[4] Bovend'Eerdt TJ, Botell RE, Wade DT. Writing SMART rehabilitation goals and achieving goal attainment scaling: a practical guide. Clin Rehabil 2009;23:352–61.

[5] Burton AK, Waddell G, Burtt R, Blair S. Patient educational material in the management of low back pain in primary care. Bull Hosp Jt Dis 1996;55:138–41.

[6] Burton AK, Waddell G, Tillotson KM, Summerton N. Information and advice to patients with back pain can have a positive effect. A randomized controlled trial of a novel educational booklet in primary care. Spine 1999;24:2484–91.

[7] Butler AC, Chapman JE, Forman EM, Beck AT. The empirical status of cognitive-behavioral therapy: a review of meta-analyses. Clin Psychol Rev 2006;26:17–31.

[8] Coia P, Morley S. Medical reassurance and patients' responses. J Psychosom Res 1998;45:377–86.

[9] Craske MG, Kircanski K, Zelikowsky M, Mystkowski J, Chowdhury N, Baker A. Optimizing inhibitory learning during exposure therapy. Behav Res Ther 2008;46:5–27.

[10] Craske MG, Rowe MK. A comparison of behavioral and cognitive treatments of phobias. In: Davey GCL, editor. Phobias: a handbook of theory, research and treatment. Chichester: Wiley & Sons; 1997. p. 247–80.

[11] Craske MG, Wolitzky-Taylor KB, Labus J, Wu S, Frese M, Mayer EA, Naliboff BD. A cognitive-behavioral treatment for irritable bowel syndrome using interoceptive exposure to visceral sensations. Behav Res Ther 2011;49:413–21.

[12] Crombez G, Eccleston C, Vlaeyen JWS, Vansteenwegen D, Lysens R, Eelen P. Exposure to physical movement in low back pain patients: Restricted effects of generalization. Health Psychol 2002;21:573–8.

[13] Crombez G, Vervaet L, Baeyens F, Lysens R, Eelen P. Do pain expectancies cause pain in chronic low back patients? A clinical investigation. Behav Res Ther 1996;34:919–25.

[14] Darlow B, Fullen BM, Dean S, Hurley DA, Baxter GD, Dowell A. The association between health care professional attitudes and beliefs and the attitudes and beliefs, clinical management, and outcomes of patients with low back pain: a systematic review. Eur J Pain 2012;16:3–17.

[15] de Jong JR, Vlaeyen JW, Onghena P, Cuypers C, den Hollander M, Ruijgrok J. Reduction of pain-related fear in complex regional pain syndrome type I: the application of graded exposure in vivo. Pain 2005;116:264–75.

[16] de Jong JR, Vlaeyen JW, Onghena P, Goossens ME, Geilen M, Mulder H. Fear of movement/(re)injury in chronic low back pain: education or exposure in vivo as mediator to fear reduction? Clin J Pain 2005;21:9–17.

[17] De Peuter S, Van Diest I, Vansteenwegen D, Van den Bergh O, Vlaeyen JW. Understanding fear of pain in chronic pain: interoceptive fear conditioning as a novel approach. Eur J Pain 2011;15:889–94.

[18] Flink IK, Nicholas MK, Boersma K, Linton SJ. Reducing the threat value of chronic pain: a preliminary replicated single-case study of interoceptive exposure versus distraction in six individuals with chronic back pain. Behav Res Ther 2009;47:721–8.

[19] Fordyce WE. Behavioral methods for chronic pain and illness. St. Louis: Mosby; 1976.

[20] Fordyce WE, Fowler RS, DeLateur B. An application of behavior modification technique to a problem of chronic pain. Behav Res Ther 1968;6:105–7.

[21] Goossens MEJB, Vlaeyen JWS, Portegeijs P, de Vet HCW, Weber W. Het rugboekje: patiëntenbrochure 'Omgaan met lage rugpijn' [The little back book: brochure "How to deal with low back pain"]. Tijdschrift Psychotherapie 2002;28:205–22.

[22] Goubert L, Francken G, Crombez G, Vansteenwegen D, Lysens R. Exposure to physical movement in chronic back pain patients: no evidence for generalization across different movements. Behav Res Ther 2002;40:415–29.

[23] Houben RM, Ostelo RW, Vlaeyen JW, Wolters PM, Peters M, Stomp-van den Berg SG. Health care providers' orientations towards common low back pain predict perceived harmfulness of physical activities and recommendations regarding return to normal activity. Eur J Pain 2005;9:173–83.

[24] Jensen MC, Brant-Zawadzki MN, Obuchowski N, Modic MT, Malkasian D, Ross JS. Magnetic resonance imaging of the lumbar spine in people without back pain. N Engl J Med 1994;331:69–73.

[25] Jensen MP. Enhancing motivation to change in pain treatment. In: Turk DC, Gatchel RJ, editors. Psychological approaches to pain management: a practitioner's handbook. New York: Guilford Press; 2002. p. 71–93.

94 J.W.S Vlaeyen et al.

[26] Kendall NAS, Linton SJ, Main CJ. Guide to assessing psychosocial yellow flags in acute low back pain: risk factors for long-term disability and work loss. Wellington: New Zealand: Accident Compensation Corporation; 1997.

[27] Kirk J. Cognitive-behavioural assessment. In: Hawton K, Salkovskis PM, Kirk J, DM Clark, editors. Cognitive behaviour therapy for psychiatric problems: a practical guide. Oxford: Oxford University Press; 1989. p. 13–51.

[28] Lindstrom I, Ohlund C, Eek C, Wallin L, Peterson LE, Fordyce WE, Nachemson AL. The effect of graded activity on patients with subacute low back pain: a randomized prospective clinical study with an operant-conditioning behavioral approach. Phys Ther 1992;72:279–90; discussion 291–3.

[29] Linton SJ, McCracken LM, Vlaeyen JW. Reassurance: help or hinder in the treatment of pain. Pain 2008;134:5–8.

[30] Linton SJ, Vlaeyen J, Ostelo R. The back pain beliefs of health care providers: are we fear-avoidant? J Occup Rehabil 2002;12:223–32.

[31] McDonald IG, Daly J, Jelinek VM, Panetta F, Gutman JM. Opening Pandora's box: the unpredictability of reassurance by a normal test result. BMJ 1996;313:329–32.

[32] Moore JE, Von Korff M, Cherkin D, Saunders K, Lorig K. A randomized trial of a cognitive-behavioral program for enhancing back pain self-care in a primary care setting. Pain 2000;88:145–53.

[33] Morris LD, Grimmer-Somers KA, Spottiswoode B, Louw QA. Virtual reality exposure therapy as treatment for pain catastrophizing in fibromyalgia patients: proof-of-concept study (Study Protocol). BMC Musculoskelet Disord;12:85.

[34] Moseley GL, Zalucki N, Birklein F, Marinus J, van Hilten JJ, Luomajoki H. Thinking about movement hurts: the effect of motor imagery on pain and swelling in people with chronic arm pain. Arthritis Rheum 2008;59:623–31.

[35] Philips HC. Avoidance behaviour and its role in sustaining chronic pain. Behav Res Ther 1987;25:273–9.

[36] Rachman S, Arntz AR. The overprediction and underprediction of pain. Clin Psychol Rev 1991;11:339–55.

[37] Rainville J, Bagnall D, Phalen L. Health care providers' attitudes and beliefs about functional impairments and chronic back pain. Clin J Pain 1995;11:287–95.

[38] Sanders S. Operant treatment. Back to basics. In: Turk DC, Gatchel RJ, editors. Psychological approaches to pain management: a practitioner's handbook. New York: Guilford Press; 2002.

[39] Thorn BE. Cognitive therapy for chronic pain. New York: Guilford Press; 2004.

[40] Trost Z, France CR, Thomas JS. Examination of the photograph series of daily activities (PHODA) scale in chronic low back pain patients with high and low kinesiophobia. Pain 2009;141:276–82.

[41] Turk DC, Gatchel RJ. Psychological approaches to pain management: a practitioner's handbook. New York: Guilford Press; 2002.

[42] Vlaeyen JW, de Jong J, Geilen M, Heuts PH, van Breukelen G. Graded exposure in vivo in the treatment of pain-related fear: a replicated single-case experimental design in four patients with chronic low back pain. Behav Res Ther 2001;39:151–66.

[43] Vlaeyen JW, de Jong J, Geilen M, Heuts PH, van Breukelen G. The treatment of fear of movement/(re)injury in chronic low back pain: further evidence on the effectiveness of exposure in vivo. Clin J Pain 2002;18:251–61.

[44] Wald J, Taylor S, Chiri LR, Sica C. Posttraumatic stress disorder and chronic pain arising from motor vehicle accidents: efficacy of interoceptive exposure plus trauma-related exposure therapy. Cogn Behav Ther 2010;39:104–13.

[45] Wolpe J. Psychotherapy by reciprocal inhibition. Stanford, CA: Stanford University Press; 1958.

Obstacles and Challenges

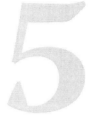

The clinical application of in vivo exposure is not always easy or success-ful. Indeed, in vivo exposure requires an impressive amount of skill to be delivered in a credible and effective way. While there are still a significant number of details that we do not know enough about to develop simple routines or decisive guidelines, there is also a substantial amount of data and considerable experience in delivering the treatment. We can therefore identify some of the obstacles and challenges that typically occur in treat-ment. In this chapter, we review the challenges that might be encountered in the application of graded in vivo exposure and suggest possible solu-tions. We focus on some of the most common challenges to delivering a psychologically based treatment for a problem that, from a patient's per-spective, is often perceived to require a biomedical solution, as well as focus on general challenges that arise when delivering a cognitive-behav-ioral treatment for fear-related problems. These challenges may become potential threats to engaging the patient in treatment and they may also affect the efficacy of the intervention. We have therefore structured this chapter in two sections. The first section deals with engaging the patient in a treatment that is not readily perceived as credible, and the second deals with a range of challenges that relate to delivering exposure in an effective fashion. As a vehicle for highlighting a selection of key challenges that clinicians might encounter, we will use the case description of a fictional

Table I
An overview of treatment challenges and solutions

Challenge	Solutions
The patient does not experience or describe their problem in terms of fear; he/she has a medical problem orientation, and exposure is not readily perceived as credible.	Teamwork: good communication between disciplines. Careful medical examination as the point of departure. A spirit of acceptance and collaboration. Ask open questions and use Socratic dialog. Personalize the rationale for treatment to closely resemble the patient's experience. Use the patient's own examples and history to convey the rationale for exposure. Use terminology that is relevant and familiar to the patient. Use didactics at the right time and in close connection to the patient's questions and worries about their pain problem and its causes.
Fear and insecurity in the therapist.	Generate experience. Improve understanding of the model. Improve understanding of (pain-related) fear and avoidance. Expose yourself to your anxiety. Role-play critical parts of the treatment and rehearse anticipated difficulties with a colleague. Use a manual and monitor adherence to the manual. Make use of supervision. Work in a team.
Fear in the patient.	Validate by reacting empathetically, but in a nonanxious manner. Model confidence through nonverbal behavior (model movements; refrain from excessive reassurance). Appropriately grade exercises to match the patient and to maximize the likelihood of success. Make it a priority to stay on track and not be diverted from the protocol of gradual, systematic, and repeated exposure to the feared movements. Balance this priority against relational issues.
Intricacies of exposure for pain-related fears: The feared outcome is unclear. The feared outcome is harm that occurs in the long term. The main concern is fear of increased pain rather than fear of harm.	Use guided discovery to elicit specific cognitions about what the feared outcome is. Develop behavioral experiments that have the possibility to correct overestimations of *probability* and *cost* of the feared outcome. Help patients to assess their reactions, and review the outcome of the experiment in terms of meaning. Use patient self-monitoring (diary) to provide objective information on levels of pain, fear, and function.

Table I
Continued

Challenge	Solutions
The avoidance is not readily apparent; it is subtle or covert (safety behaviors).	Learn to detect safety behaviors through careful observation. Address the use of safety behaviors explicitly, and make elimination of the use of safety behaviors a joint effort together with the patient.
Despite high scores during assessment, the patient displays low avoidance behavior during exposure.	Investigate whether low avoidance is due to safety behaviors. Reconsider whether exposure treatment is the appropriate treatment of choice. Investigate the significance of coexisting problems that may make the intervention more difficult or less likely to succeed.
While the patient gradually improves, he/she expresses cognitions that signal learning of exceptions to the general rule that certain movements cause damage to the back.	Keep in mind that by performing a restricted number of activities, the patient may learn that there are exceptions to the general rule that movements may cause damage to the back. Actively work toward generalization by practicing exposure in many different situations, especially home situations and daily activities that are typical for the patient.

patient, Robert, who underwent exposure treatment with an unsuccessful outcome. Whereas this case is fictional, it is based on experience with some of the less successful in vivo exposure treatments we have performed. It touches on several issues that relate to engagement, as well as to the intricacies of graded in vivo exposure for patients with pain-related fear. In relation to the challenges that can be encountered, we will introduce possible solutions as well as outline competencies needed to successfully perform this treatment. Table I provides a short overview of the challenges and solutions that will be addressed in this chapter. We conclude the chapter with an overview of competencies that we consider to be prerequisites for the effective delivery of in vivo exposure for pain-related fear.

Case Description

Robert was a 48-year-old data consultant. He had back pain that had waxed and waned since he was in his twenties. About every third month, he had a bout of low back pain that kept him bedridden for approximately a week. The aftermath of such a bout lasted for weeks, and he described his recovery as getting slower and slower as the years went by. He had been treated by a physiotherapist and followed a special exercise regimen. He had also visited a chiropractor on a regular basis. He described being careful not to make any sudden movements when doing his exercise program so as to not provoke the pain. He had sought the advice of a primary care physician several times when he had felt stiffness in his back, which for Robert was sign of impending trouble. A thorough physical check-up, including magnetic resonance imaging, had indicated that there was no underlying pathology that required biomedical attention. Although Robert had been told that his back pain was quite common and benign, he remained very worried and described the pain as excruciating, at times. During his last visit, his primary care physician asked him to fill out a battery of questionnaires to get a broader picture of his pain experience and the consequences it had for him.

Robert's scores showed that he was quite sure that his pain was caused by physical damage and that "worn-out disks" meant that he needed to be careful when performing strenuous movements involving his back muscles. Because his pain problem was worsening, Robert believed that the disk problem may have become worse due to some unexpected and ill-considered heavy lifting that he had recently performed. Robert said that it was important for him to find ways to prevent pain episodes because he was concerned about becoming permanently disabled if things continued to develop. He described a preference for a longer-term contact with a physiotherapist who could provide him with ergonomic tips for avoiding unnecessary back strain. However, his primary care physician referred him to the primary care center's health psychologist. She was a specialist in pain with experience in graded in vivo exposure. Robert hesitated but complied because he considered it worth a try.

During their first meeting, the health psychologist performed the assessment as described in detail in Chapter 3. The Photograph Series of Daily Activities (PHODA; see Table II for details) showed that Robert tended to avoid movements and activities involving bending and lifting and movements that implicate compression of the spine such as jumping and running. After completion of the assessment procedure, the psychologist integrated the identified beliefs, thoughts, feelings, and behaviors into a personalized fear-avoidance model (see Fig. 1 for details). She carefully reviewed this model with Robert, as described in Chapter 4. During the review, Robert was relatively quiet, but he seemed to accept the reformulation of his pain problem as presented by the health psychologist. The rationale for in vivo exposure was provided, and personal goals were developed. Thereafter, the hierarchy for exposure was developed and the first session of exposure scheduled. At the first exposure session, Robert and the psychologist worked together and agreed on starting with movement involving bending of the back, with the ultimate goal of being able to lift a crate of beer bottles from the floor without hesitation or safety behaviors.

During the exposure trials at the initial levels of the hierarchy, Robert described the experiments as "not really a problem" to do. He expected a moderate increase in pain while working through the hierarchy, but this pain did not signify damage. He was able to successfully pick up

Table II
Fear hierarchy for Robert

Fear Hierarchy	PHODA Item
100	Lift a crate of bottles
	Jump off a stool
	Dig in the garden
80	Run in the woods
	Do car repair work
	Run downstairs
60	Do vacuum cleaning
	Twist and turn the back
	Bend forward
	Lift groceries out of the car
40	Bend over to tie shoelaces
	Lift grocery bags
20	Squat down
	Turn over in bed

Abbreviation: PHODA, Photograph Series of Daily Activities.

a pen from a chair and then pick it up from the floor. The moderate pain increases that he expected while performing the movements were confirmed by his experience. The psychologist noticed that he performed the movements in a controlled way and that he braced his back. She discussed this observation with Robert, and thereafter he appeared to try to consciously let go of some of the control while performing the movements. He experienced no increase in pain after this time but did not consider this experience to be meaningful in helping him to understand his back pain. After this experience, Robert and the psychologist jointly decided to go to the next level of the hierarchy, which involved lifting. Starting with an empty crate, Robert responded in a similar way, with no specific expectation of damage or relevant pain increase before the exposure. As he progressed up the hierarchy by gradually adding beer bottles to the crate, Robert started to hesitate. He reported that it was "getting too heavy now" and worried that the lift would trigger a severe bout of pain and that he would be bedridden the following day. He described that he thought that there was "something not right" with his back and that the lift might result in an intensely painful reaction. He judged the likelihood that this would happen as 50%, but if he were to repeat the lift 10 times, the likelihood would go up considerably. The psychologist asked to what

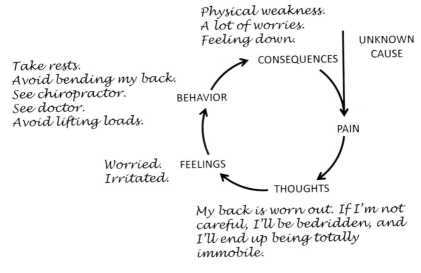

Fig. 1. Fear-avoidance cycle for Robert.

degree the likelihood would increase, but Robert was adamant that he could not tell other than "just a lot." Robert found it difficult to be explicit about the expected pain increase and said that it would be "really bad." He complied with lifting the crate repeatedly up to 10 times to test his expectancies and performed the 10 lifts without incident, although the psychologist noticed that Robert was tense, held his breath, and braced his back while lifting. Afterward, he reported that his pain increased moderately but that it "went better than I expected." Robert and the psychologist jointly decided to end the session, and homework was planned, for which Robert agreed to repeat the same movements as performed during the session at home (10 lifts, 3 times a day).

Robert did not attend his next session. The psychologist called him, and Robert said that a few days after the session he had a serious bout of back pain. He was reluctant to talk, but did say that "it was of course really dumb to provoke this." He refused further participation in the treatment and questioned its validity for his problem. He said that he had sought advice from another health care professional who confirmed that bending and lifting were very unwise to do with his type of problem. The psychologist offered a joint meeting together with the primary care physiotherapist, but Robert declined, and the contact was terminated.

Challenges Related to Treatment Credibility and Engagement

One aspect that is noticeable in Robert's presentation is his medical problem orientation. Evidence can be seen in his history of seeking medically oriented solutions and his hesitation when referred to the psychologist. This situation is not unusual, many patients come to us with a host of beliefs, attitudes, and ideas about their problem. Their thoughts and beliefs often center on medical explanations for why they are suffering pain, and expectations of biomedically oriented solutions are therefore plausible. Medical orientation is closely related with pain-related fear and avoidance. Almost without exception, patients come to treatment with a predominantly medical model and problem definition [2]. In addition, Robert is just one of many who have attempted to treat their pain in a large variety of ways with limited or no success. This effort usually encompasses home remedies, consultations with nonprofessionals, consultations with complementary medical professionals, and consultations with a range of health care professionals. Consequently, it is not surprising that a patient might be skeptical about a new treatment, especially if it does not coincide with his or her own conceptualization of the problem. Indeed, patients in general might not fully understand or accept in vivo exposure as a credible treatment option. Consider for example, that in two studies, exposure was the treatment least preferred by patients [3; Linton, in preparation], and randomized controlled trials of treatment (see Chapter 8 for a review) report a significant number of dropouts, ranging from 30% to 58% [6,7,14], which might signal a lack of perceived clinical relevance by patients.

This initial lack of clinical validity might lead to difficulties, whereby the patient does not understand or accept the idea of exposure. Their concerns may be expressed in the form of verbal comments, nonverbal behaviors, or in the form of more subtle changes in responsiveness while communicating during assessment or treatment. These variations in the expression of doubt and skepticism require a degree of skill on the part of the therapist in attending to the subtleties of the interaction to detect and respond to these issues in an appropriate way. It is better to gently probe the patient indirectly when they express uncertainty rather than simply to ignore one's own suspicion that they are experiencing doubt. Tentative empathetic reflection, for example, "So you're not too sure about whether this is for you?" is a tried and tested way of facilitating further engagement before asking more direct questions about whether the patient finds this treatment to be desirable and credible.

For many patients, careful assessment and provision of information will promote perceived credibility and engagement. In the case of Robert, the treatment was performed by a health psychologist with competence in cognitive-behavioral therapy (CBT). Even though she was both knowledgeable and competent, there was an obvious mismatch between the therapist's and Robert's expectancies about appropriateness of conceptualization and treatment. For Robert, the psychologist lacked basic credibility in dealing with his pain problem. Indeed, for patients who are strongly convinced of a biomedical cause for their pain complaints, being referred to a psychologist may be perceived as invalidating, because it may suggest that their pain is judged to be psychogenic. This issue is of course not unique to the treatment of pain-related fear, and most psychologists and those working within a psychological framework will have encountered the problem of engagement with patients who retain a strong biomedical orientation. In most circumstances, an exploration of how pain has influenced the patient's life and well-being will be sufficient to introduce the idea that even when there is a known physical cause for the pain, there are multiple, complex, downstream psychological effects. It is often easy to demonstrate that these effects are influenced by factors other than the original cause of the pain, for example mood, and that the individual's response to the pain experience may be just as important as the cause. This demonstration is often sufficient to address the common misconception that the absence of biomedical pathology means that the pain is imagined.

To circumvent and resolve these potential difficulties, there is an advantage in delivering this type of treatment in the context of a team that includes a CBT-competent physiotherapist and psychologist. Moreover, it may be advantageous to initiate the assessment procedure with a highly credible and thorough medical examination, for example by a general practitioner, rehabilitation physician, or orthopedic surgeon, even if there is no apparent question regarding a medical diagnosis and the presence of pathology.

Given the potential mismatch between the patient's initial model and the model on which exposure is based, a high level of competency is needed to set the stage for successful engagement in exposure. A carefully conducted case conceptualization and rationale may promote perceived credibility and engagement. Although Robert's therapist appears to have accomplished this goal, we note that Robert's quiet demeanor and easy acceptance of the formulation might not have indicated assent but rather a reluctance to engage in confrontation with a "powerful" health professional, whom he might not wish to alienate. Alternatively, he may have decided that to satisfy the referring general practitioner, he would go through the motions of treatment simply to demonstrate that it did not work and to get further access to more traditional physical treatments.

Although Chapter 4 provides the basic knowledge necessary to conduct exposure treatment, it requires training and supervision to acquire the skills to draw on this knowledge and to integrate the aspects that arise in the assessment into a patient-specific, fear-avoidance model that is recognized and accepted by the patient. Patients usually do not experience or express their pain problem in terms of fear or fear avoidance beliefs and behaviors. For example, Robert said that he was very worried about back pain and described it as, at times, excruciating. He did not, however, express or frame his experience in a way that made it easy to recognize fear-avoidance beliefs and behaviors, their interrelations, and their effects on the development and maintenance of his pain problem. Whereas a standardized assessment procedure, such as laid out in Chapter 3, is a helpful tool, the therapist also needs to draw on their general knowledge of cognitive and behavioral aspects of emotion so that they can recognize a patient's key cognitions and overt and covert behaviors and the potential effect of these on the development and maintenance of the pain problem.

Based on a thorough assessment, the therapist needs to be able to build an individualized fear-avoidance model that indicates potential targets for intervention and can be used to convey the treatment rationale to the patient in a credible way. In fact, successful engagement of patients in the intervention is most likely when the therapist has the skill to help patients see the potential relevance of the fear-avoidance model in relation to their own history of difficulties. Whereas direct questions can be asked about whether patients see the pain-related fear mechanisms in their own case, and whether the description of avoidance fits their case, this goal is best achieved via active collaboration and a tailor-made treatment rationale. This rationale is usually promoted by applying specific and concrete examples of the relation between pain and the thoughts, feelings, and behaviors that the patient has disclosed during the assessment. It is important to present the formulation in language that is familiar to the patient rather than using unfamiliar technical terminology.

Finally, making use of didactic teaching might be a helpful addition if carefully timed and prepared (see Dialog Boxes 1 and 2 from Chapter 4). This strategy can be used to correct obvious biomedical misconceptions, to explain how pain might persist without pathology, and to illustrate how biology and psychology may interplay to give a fuller understanding of pain and its effects. However, especially with patients such as Robert, who have doubts about the usefulness of in vivo exposure, it is important to promote active collaboration and to refrain from being overly directive when providing the rationale. Being overly directive could lead to a situation in which a mismatch of models and lack of trust and perceived credibility remain hidden under the surface, eventually leading to resistance and drop out.

The case of Robert highlights credibility and engagement challenges that eventually led him to drop out of treatment. However, obstacles are sometimes more subtle and may challenge the efficacy of the treatment. The next section deals with common issues that may arise when performing exposure and links them to some of the important competencies required by the therapist.

Challenges to Delivering Exposure: Staying on Track

In general, exposure treatment for anxiety-related problems is demanding for patients and therapists. Patients often display high levels of distress when confronted with anxiety-provoking stimuli, which can generate uncertainty, anxiety, and insecurity in the therapist, causing the therapist to drift away from or avoid the prescribed steps laid out in the manual [13]. It has been shown that fear-avoidance beliefs are also present in clinicians treating patients with pain, and these are related to a reorientation toward medical problem solving [1,5,8]. These factors increase the risk of diverting from the treatment approach outlined in this book. Although a thorough medical examination may resolve many of the therapist's concerns, when it comes to the risk of the patient being (re)injured during exposure, there will always remain some ambiguity and uncertainty regarding the presence of biomedical factors that may contribute to the pain problem. Special training and supervision is required to be able to consistently model non-fearful behavior, regardless of the level of distress displayed by the patient.

Common challenges to deal with during exposure treatment are pain flare-ups. Pain flare-ups can be distressing for many patients and therapists and, as in the case of Robert, can challenge engagement and jeopardize adherence to the protocol. There are several ways of dealing with pain flare-ups that can counteract or prevent the risk of patient dis-engagement. First, empathy and validation of the patient's experience is a prerequisite for a trusting relationship, and the therapist needs to use clinical judgment to balance adherence to the fear-avoidance model and treatment protocol against the need to attend to any relational issues that might present themselves. The therapist also needs to refrain from exces-sive reassurance, while responding empathetically, when confronted with distress. For example, if pain increases during or after an exposure session, the patient might be convinced that (re)injury occurred and that there is a need for renewed medical investigation or a radical change in treat-ment strategy (for example stopping or decreasing the activity demands). At such times, the therapist should try to estimate the cause of the pain increase without conveying alarm. If the pain expression is different from before, and the patient shows symptoms suggestive of a biomedical cause (for example, loss of bowel or bladder control, fever, weight loss, loss of strength in the legs), new diagnostic tests should be carried out. However, such symptoms are extraordinarily rare, and it is unlikely that they will be encountered. In most cases, a more likely alternative explanation for the pain is available. Increased pain is most often a result of the re-engagement of muscles that have been relatively neglected or the effect of exercise on the muscles, or the patient may have engaged in anticipatory tensing of the muscles before executing the item on the hierarchy.

Distress due to pain flare-ups can be managed proactively by at-tempting to alter the patient's expectations and to reduce the likelihood of catastrophizing. For example, pain flare-ups can be made predictable by explicitly generating the expectation of pain increase before exposure ("It is not uncommon to experience pain flare-ups during the days after this session"). When explaining the rationale for treatment, pain flare-ups can be normalized as an integral part of treatment rather than a signal of impending treatment failure. Lastly, a pain flare-up can be reframed as a good preparation for relapse prevention because it allows the patient to prepare for pain increases that will probably occur during the post-treatment period ("It is good that this happened now, so we can find new ways to deal with the pain flare-ups that you might experience later on"). Overall, the goal is to design the exposure exercises in such a way that they will elicit a fear response but will also have a positive outcome in terms of new learning. This requires balancing progression through the hierarchy between moving forward and repetition, depending on the verbal and nonverbal feedback the patient provides. Our experience indicates that if an initial pain fluctuation can be dealt with successfully, pain-related fears will decrease quickly, and subsequent pain increases will generate less concern.

In vivo exposure exercises and behavior experiments do not imply that patients are exposed to any stimulus. The activities that patients are exposed to are reasonable and safe for everyone, consist of common movements that people perform in everyday life and that were part of the patient's own behavioral repertoire before injury, and preferably help the patient re-engage with valued life goals. In addition, engagement in exposure can be enhanced by carefully outlining subsequent steps and by modeling the movements, thereby conveying the message that the movements are safe. Indeed, it can be difficult to motivate patients to perform an activity or a movement that in their experience and belief is harmful for their back. Starting with relatively nonthreatening activities, patients may experience increased confidence in the approach and that their (catastrophic) beliefs are incorrect. To achieve this goal, the therapist learns to collaborate with the patient to ensure that the exposure is gradual, systematic, repeated and prolonged and to be able to predict, identify, and address problems.

Challenges to Delivering Exposure: Intricacies of Exposure for Pain-Related Fear

Exposure using behavioral experiments requires that patients verbalize a specific expectation of what the feared outcome (propositional knowledge) is in terms of what they do, for example, "If I bend, then my spinal nerve will break." Initially, the patient may not have such a specific expectation, and a common answer is that the patient just expects an increase in pain. It is the task of the therapist to investigate the personal meaning of such a pain increase, which requires a high level of proficiency. For example, in the case of Robert, there appeared to have been difficulties arriving at joint and explicit expectations about the outcome ("a lot" more pain) and its meaning ("That would be really bad") when conducting the challenging lifting experiments. The therapist needs to develop the ability to elicit, via guided discovery, specific cognitions about what the feared outcome is, as well as the ability to help patients assess their reactions and review the outcome of an experiment in terms of meaning.

An initial nonspecific answer to the question of expectation during or after exposure may, after further questioning, reveal a specific damage expectation, but the expectation and fear of increased pain, rather than fear of harm, are often present. Moreover, sometimes the feared consequence is harm that may occur not immediately but rather in the long-term ("If the pain feels like this, I might become handicapped and bedridden in the future"). These expectations of delayed catastrophe require that the therapist develop the skill to design behavioral experiments that provide the opportunity to correct this overestimate as well as its cost, not only in the short-term but also in the long-term. Systematic use of a diary, in which the patients tracks the relationship between pain, fear, and function, can be very helpful in correcting catastrophic expectations and memory biases related to these fears.

In principle, Robert fulfilled all of the formal criteria for being a good candidate for exposure treatment. He scored high on common standardized measures such as the Tampa Scale for Kinesiophobia (TSK) and the Pain Catastrophizing Scale (PCS), and with the PHODA, he identified a range of movements and activities that he considered harmful to his back. He also reported worry and the fear that the pain signaled damage to his back. However, it is not uncommon that the assessment picture is more ambiguous and more difficult to interpret. In addition, the patient may progress through the fear hierarchy without any apparent difficulty, despite high scores on standardized, pain-related fear measures such as the TSK. Furthermore, pain-related fear is just one part of a complex problem in the context of multiple psychological and social problems. These variations can make it difficult to decide whether the individual is a good candidate for graded in vivo exposure. The assessment procedures and recommendations that are provided in Chapter 3 are based mainly on published studies and correlational research and may not directly reflect an individual patient in the clinic. The clinical assessment and selection procedure is designed to help optimize the fit between the patient's needs and the best possible treatment. As with any other assessment, this procedure is not an exact science. Observing actual avoidance behavior is one good method of determining whether the patient is appropriate for exposure. Unfortunately, there are no standardized techniques yet available to assess behavioral avoidance. However, you can ask the patient to perform movements or activities that most patients with similar pain problems find threatening. Make sure that the patient engages in the movement to the point of avoidance rather than simply describing the problem. This strategy is helpful in ascertaining whether fear is present and whether the patient is actually avoiding. What might happen if the treatment is offered, but the patient is not actually avoiding? As far as we know, in vivo exposure treatment has no negative effects if given to someone without pain-related fear, and the assessment glitch should become obvious very quickly. For example, a patient at our clinic fulfilled all of the usual criteria for treatment. However, when we started the exposure, she was able to do all of the elements in the hierarchy during the first session with little fear, provoked pain, or problem. During the exposure session, it became clear that exposure was not going to be helpful and that the problem might instead focus on the workplace. A basic competency required for performing this treatment is the ability to assess the significance of coexisting problems that might make the intervention more difficult or less likely to succeed such as depression, heavy use of pain medication, significant work related issues, or insurance issues.

Sometimes patients progress through the fear hierarchy without any obvious avoidance, while at the same time, their self-report signals that they have not changed their fear and avoidance cognitions. In such cases, patients could be engaging in subtle forms of avoidance in the form of inadvertent or unconscious safety-seeking behaviors [9,10] such as mental distraction, bracing the back or neck, holding their breath, clenching their teeth, slowing down or speeding up their movements, or making excessive use of the leg muscles. These behaviors can inhibit the purpose of exposure and the ability to receive corrective information during the experiment. Other examples include lifting ergonomically, supporting the back with a hand, or wearing a corset. Patients use these safety-seeking behaviors to avoid frightening events that may occur. In this way, performance of an activity does not lead to the desired decrease in anxiety or correction of catastrophic thinking because the patient learns that the activity can be carried

Table III
Overview of competencies required for graded in vivo exposure for pain-related fear

Prerequisites

1) Knowledge of how learning theory applies to behaviors displayed by patients with pain and pain-related fear. Knowledge of the ways people respond behaviorally to pain as a threat and how this may perpetuate or worsen the pain problem.

2) Specific knowledge of the role of safety behaviors, their function, and their consequences.

3) Knowledge of how cognitive theories apply to patients with pain-related fear, with a specific focus on the roles of fear-avoidance beliefs, catastrophizing, and expectancies.

4) Knowledge of relevant measures for pain-related fear and avoidance and the ability to interpret these measures and to integrate them into the intervention; knowledge of self-monitoring, as well as the ability to integrate and make full use of self-monitoring within the intervention. For example, can self-monitoring be used to provide objective information on the levels of pain and function for patients who are very fearful of delayed pain flare-ups and disability while at home between exposure sessions?

5) Ability to model non–pain-related fear behavior, such as by modeling movements, refraining from excessive reassurance, and reacting empathetically, without mirroring distress, when confronted with pain flare-ups and other issues that may worry the patient.

6) Ability to use clinical judgment to balance adherence to the fear-avoidance model and treatment protocol against the need to attend to any relational issues that may present themselves.

Skills During Assessment and Engagement in Treatment

7) Ability to draw on knowledge of (safety-seeking) behaviors and cognition to identify key cognitions and overt and covert behaviors, their interrelations, and their effect on the development and maintenance of the patient's pain problem.

8) Ability to integrate these aspects into a personalized fear-avoidance model that provides potential targets for intervention using graded in vivo exposure, and ability to collaborate with the patient to see the potential relevance of the fear-avoidance model to his or her own difficulties.

9) Ability to explain the rationale for targeting avoided and potentially painful movements and activities with graded exposure.

Skills During Intervention

10) Ability to develop behavioral experiments in accordance with the fear hierarchy and the patient's personal goals, which may help the patient to gradually become exposed to the feared stimuli, and to test the validity of the patient's assumptions and beliefs about performing specific feared movements and activities.

Table III
Continued

11) Ability to work with the patient to ensure that the exposure to movements and activities is gradual, systematic, repeated, and prolonged and to be able to identify problems. That is, the ability to plan experiments that will elicit a fear response but will also likely have a positive outcome, and to balance progression through the hierarchy between moving forward and repetition, depending on learning as well as relational issues.

12) Ability to develop behavioral experiments that can correct overestimations of the *probability* and *cost* of the feared outcome. This includes the ability to elicit, via guided discovery, specific cognitions about what the feared outcome is, and the ability to help patients assess their reactions and review the outcome of the experiment in terms of meaning.

13) Ability (to help the patient) to identify and circumvent any covert avoidance (such as mental distraction) or use of safety-seeking behaviors (such as bracing the back or neck, holding one's breath, clenching one's teeth, slowing down or speeding up, excessive use of leg muscles) so that the patient can obtain the maximum amount of corrective information during the experiment.

out with the use of a safety-seeking behavior. The fact that the catastrophe will not occur is basically attributed to the use of the safety-seeking behavior. In the short-term anxiety decreases, but in the long-term, pain-related fear is maintained. In such cases, the exposure exercise can be repeated without engaging in the safety-seeking behavior. The use and detection of safety-seeking behaviors may also be dealt with explicitly and in collaboration with the patient during the preparatory phase of treatment. This joint effort provides the opportunity to detect and let go of any safety-seeking behaviors that might counteract the extinction of fear.

Lastly, as therapy progresses, it becomes important to focus on generalization. If only a limited number of situations are included in exposure therapy, there is a risk that the newly learned thoughts and behaviors and the reduction in fear will not generalize to new situations. By performing a restricted number of activities and movements, the patient might learn that there are exceptions to the rule that "certain movements cause damage to the back" instead of learning the new rule that "back load movements do not cause damage to the spine" [4]. Therefore, it is important to be aware of expressions that might signal learning an exception to the rule (e.g., "I can do more than I thought"). Practicing exposure in as many different situations as possible, especially home situations and daily activities that are typical for the patient, will enhance the generalization of fear extinction.

Competencies Required for Graded In Vivo Exposure for Pain-Related Fear

The challenges addressed above relate to the intricacy of performing a psychologically based treatment for a problem that, from a patient perspective, is often perceived to require a biomedical solution, and also relate to the challenges that arise when performing a cognitive-behavioral treatment for a fear-related problem. Graded in vivo exposure for patients with pain and high levels of pain-related fear requires thorough knowledge of the psychology of pain, as well as general and specific competencies in the application of CBT. As with any treatment manual for CBT, the chapters in this book address most of the competencies required to achieve a level of outcome success equivalent to that in published studies. Drawing on the extensive overview of competency requirements for the delivery of effective CBT for anxiety and depressive disorders published by the United Kingdom Department of Health [11,12], we have selected and adapted those CBT competencies that specifically apply to in vivo exposure treatment with behavioral experiments for pain-related fear. Whereas most of these competencies are already detailed in the above case, Table III provides a structured overview of the knowledge and skills required to increase the likelihood of a successful outcome of graded in vivo exposure for pain-related fear. Note that we do not address general CBT competencies that relate to the ability to structure sessions, monitor and promote the collaborative nature of sessions, help patients generate relevant goals, adhere to an agreed-upon agenda, or plan and review relevant and well-tailored homework assignments, as these are prerequisites.

References

[1]   Coudeyre E, Rannou F, Tubach F, Baron G, Coriat F, Brin S, Revel M, Poiraudeau S. General practitioners' fear-avoidance beliefs influence their management of patients with low back pain. Pain 2006;124:330–7.
[2]   Eccleston C, Crombez G. Worry and chronic pain: a misdirected problem solving model. Pain 2007;132:233–6.

[3]   George SZ, Robinson ME. Preference, expectation, and satisfaction in a clinical trial of behavioral interventions for acute and sub-acute low back pain. J Pain 2010;11:1074–82.

[4]   Goubert L, Francken G, Crombez G, Vansteenwegen D, Lysens R. Exposure to physical movement in chronic back pain patients: no evidence for generalization across different movements. Behav Res Ther 2002;40:415–29.

[5]   Houben RM, Ostelo RW, Vlaeyen JW, Wolters PM, Peters M, Stomp-van den Berg SG. Health care providers' orientations towards common low back pain predict perceived harmfulness of physical activities and recommendations regarding return to normal activity. Eur J Pain 2005;9:173–83.

[6]   Leeuw M, Goossens ME, van Breukelen GJ, de Jong JR, Heuts PH, Smeets RJ, Koke AJ, Vlaeyen JW. Exposure in vivo versus operant graded activity in chronic low back pain patients: results of a randomized controlled trial. Pain 2008;138:192–207.

[7]   Linton SJ, Boersma K, Jansson M, Overmeer T, Lindblom K, Vlaeyen JW. A randomized controlled trial of exposure in vivo for patients with spinal pain reporting fear of work-related activities. Eur J Pain 2008;12:722–30.

[8]   Linton SJ, McCracken LM, Vlaeyen JW, Linton SJ, McCracken LM, Vlaeyen JWS. Reassurance: help or hinder in the treatment of pain. Pain 2008;134:5–8.

[9]   Milosevic I, Radomsky AS. Safety behaviour does not necessarily interfere with exposure therapy. Behav Res Ther 2008;46:1111–8.

[10] Rachman S, Radomsky AS, Shafran R. Safety behaviour: a reconsideration. Behav Res Ther 2008;46:163–73.

[11] Roth A, Pilling S. The competences required to deliver effective cognitive and behavioural therapy for people with depression and with anxiety disorders. In: Publications policy and guidance. U.K. Department of Health; 2007. Available at: http://www.dh.gov.uk/en/publicationsandstatistics/publications/publicationspolicyandguidance/DH_078537.

[12] Roth AD, Pilling S. Using an evidence-based methodology to identify the competences required to deliver effective cognitive and behavioural therapy for depression and anxiety disorders. Behav Cogn Psychother 2008;36:129–47.

[13] Waller G. Evidence-based treatment and therapist drift. Behav Res Ther 2009;47:119–27.

[14] Woods MP, Asmundson GJ. Evaluating the efficacy of graded in vivo exposure for the treatment of fear in patients with chronic back pain: a randomized controlled clinical trial. Pain 2008;136:271–80.

Evaluating Graded Exposure
as a Treatment

6

In this and the next two chapters, we review the current evidence for the efficacy of the graded exposure protocol described in Chapter 4. Several other authors have used the fear-avoidance model in treatment, but they have not used the protocol described here, and we consider their studies in Chapter 9. This chapter outlines the strategy we have used and examines the conceptual relationship between the single-case series and randomized controlled trials (RCTs) reported in the next chapters. Although single-case methodology is well established in certain areas of behavioral change, it is less well known in the study of pain treatments, and this chapter provides a review of the methodology and explicitly links it to RCTs.

Randomized Controlled Trials Versus Single-Case Series

In the hierarchy of evidence for judging the effectiveness of treatments, RCTs are acknowledged as superior to case studies because, in principle, RCTs are able to control for more potential sources of bias. Nevertheless, *experimental* single case studies are capable of establishing the likely effectiveness of treatments. Both types of study attempt to control for several possible alternative rival hypotheses [5] that could explain changes in the outcome measures caused by events other than the effect of treatment.

These threats to the validity of studies include the following. (1) *History*: the possibility that an event unrelated to treatment coincides with treatment and is sufficient to cause change. (2) *Maturation*: the possibly that if the problem were left untreated, it would improve of its own accord. The term maturation refers to developmental change usually associated with early phases of the lifespan, and "spontaneous remission" has been used as the corresponding term with regard to disease and dysfunction. (3) *Regression to the mean*: refers to a statistical phenomenon related to the inherently less than perfect reliability of measurement. The unreliability of measurement means that repeated measurements for a given patient will differ. If the patient's initial score is toward the extreme of the scale, the repeated measure will most likely be toward the mean value of the scale [3]. (4) *Measurement*: refers to the effect of repeated exposure to the measure itself. This effect is most obvious with regard to tests of cognitive ability, where repetition of an item will help the person learn the correct answer. (5) *Instrumentation*: similar to measurement but refers to a change in the measurement properties of the measuring instrument. This is readily illustrated by the example of a 30-cm long metal ruler. The length of the ruler is determined by the ambient temperature. Thus, when the ruler is at 0°C, it will measure an object held at a constant temperature as longer than when the ruler is at 25°C. The equivalent phenomenon is perhaps more difficult to conceptualize in psychometric terms, but it is widespread. For example, an individual's subjective appreciation of wine changes following exposure to a wine tasting lesson. There is evidence that the perceptual experience of the unpleasantness of pain varies as a function of exposure to it [13]. Randomized controlled trials routinely control for all of these threats to validity and also for others related to well-known nonspecific factors such as the expectation of treatment gain and measurement biases attributable to the observer (data collector). When an RCT is well designed, it may also control for other critical features relating to the therapist, for example, equivalence of therapist competence in two treatment arms. These classes of events have been extensively discussed in relation to both RCTs and single-case studies [9,12].

The left side of Fig. 1 schematizes a sequence of measures that take place in evaluating a therapy (assessment → pretreatment → posttreatment → follow-up) and includes what we refer to as different levels of measurement. These levels are distinguished by two features: first, the frequency and timing of measurement and second, the focus of the measure. The latter is also often associated with the psychometric properties of the scales. Measures at the standard/global level generally assess constructs such as disability, interference, catastrophizing, depression, and anxiety. These are the familiar focus of many RCTs of cognitive-behavioral therapy (CBT) for chronic pain. In essence, each measure attempts to assess a sample of items that are regarded as good representations of the construct. The development of such measures, frequently questionnaires, follows a standardized procedure. In the initial stages, many items thought to represent the construct are collated and administered to a large sample of individuals. The statistical analyses have two general aims: to select items with suitable psychometric properties (dispersion of means and homogeneity of variation) and to select items that show intercorrelation coefficients of sufficient magnitude. Items that are too highly correlated are essentially redundant because they share too much in common, and a choice must be made to exclude one of the pair. Items that show low intercorrelations with other items are also discarded because they are

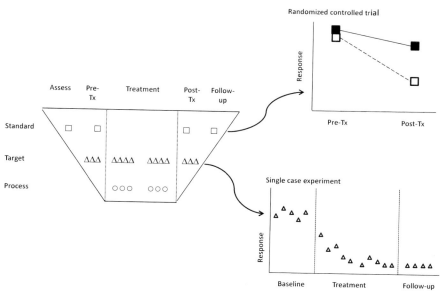

Fig. 1. Measurement and the link between randomized controlled trials and experimental single-case studies.

clearly not a good representation of the construct. It may take several iterations to achieve a working measure that is then administered, along with other established measures, to different groups in order to establish its construct validity, that is, to produce evidence that the measure correlates with measures that it is predicted to correlate with and does not correlate with measures for which a relationship is not expected. This strategy is designed to select a set of items with common variance that captures the construct in general. The measure thus aims to assess some aspect of the construct that is relevant to some degree for most people.

Whereas this strategy works well for the population at large and produces construct validity, the development strategy deliberately ignores items that might be very important to an individual and which might be the specific focus of treatment. For example, the items of the Roland-Morris Disability Questionnaire (RDQ) have general relevance but may not sample the exact behavioral limitations of a particular individual. The pursuit of psychometrically reliable measures with good construct validity often comes at a cost when it comes to measuring specific complaints or features that are relevant to an individual. From the perspective of the individual, the items that have been discarded might represent perfectly one's experience of the problem; in the parlance of psychometrics, such items have high criterion validity. This distinction will be illustrated with regard to behavioral activity in our discussion of the single-case series. Standard/global measures are not particularly suitable for the study of individuals because they do not necessarily tap criterion measures. In addition, they are not designed for repeated administration over a short period of time and are often too lengthy. For the purpose of studying an individual intensively over time, we need to construct measures of outcomes that capture the individual's *target* complaints and/or processes that are deemed essential to the therapy; these are shown in the second level of Fig. 1.

There is a range of sophisticated measurement technology from the field of applied behavior analysis, in which single-case studies have been used as the preferred method for investigating the application of behavior change methods [4,8]. In the series of case studies examined in this chapter, we have used a daily diary that includes items selected from established questionnaires designed to measure the three key cognitive components of the fear-avoidance model: fear of movement/(re)injury, fear of pain, and catastrophizing. The model states that a successful intervention will reduce the strength with which an individual holds these beliefs. We therefore expected that these target beliefs would change when graded exposure treatment was introduced. In addition to measuring these three core beliefs, we have routinely measured the daily experience of pain, although the fear-avoidance model does not explicitly suggest that the experience of pain will change during treatment. In contrast, the fear-avoidance model indicates that the behavioral repertoire of the individual should change as a result of treatment. In some of the latter studies, we performed indirect assessments of behavioral activity with an accelerometer to measure general behavioral activity. Participants also nominated specific behaviors of high value to them and recorded their success in accomplishing these on a daily basis. In contrast to the standard/global measures, the psychometric properties of many target measures are less well defined. When the target is an observable behavior, it is possible to assess whether raters agree on its occurrence. With measures of beliefs, such as those used in the case series reported here, the stability of the measure during the baseline period, when the expectation is of no change, may be regarded as an extensive examination of its test-retest stability.

In the context of single-case studies, the *process* level in Fig. 1 refers to observations on changes and critical events within treatment sessions. For example, we might monitor an individual's reported level of fear during exposure to a feared stimulus, or we might assess the strength of beliefs about possible outcomes during a behavioral experiment. Details from this type of process measure are rarely reported in published reports, irrespective of whether they are single cases or RCTs, yet paradoxically they may be among the most frequent measures used by active clinicians. We simply note that we have little published information at this level of analysis.

As shown in Fig. 1, RCTs use global/standard measures to capture representative data from many participants. The simplest design, illustrated in the upper right of the figure, requires that measures be taken on two occasions, before and after treatment (better trials will include a measure taken at follow-up). Assuming that participants are randomly allocated to the treatment and control arms of the trial, the pretreatment measures are expected to be equivalent, and the crucial test of the effect of the treatment lies in the comparison of the two groups at the end of treatment (and follow-up). In this basic design, a control group can effectively rule out major alternative plausible accounts for the change: maturation, history, regression to the mean, instrumentation, and biases concerned with the selection of participants. Well-designed RCTs with certain types of control groups will also be able to control for other plausible hypotheses related to placebo effects, the expectation of receiving an effective treatment, and the characteristics of the therapist.

Single-case experiments may also include measurements at the standard/global level, but in the absence of a control group, changes between pre- and posttreatment measurements cannot be easily interpreted, for example, we do not know whether the changes are part of a natural fluctuation that would have occurred without the intervening treatment. Single-case experiments overcome the limitations of a restricted number of measurement occasions in two ways: by designing the study so that more frequent observations are taken, and wherever possible, randomizing the point in time when treatment starts. Randomizing the occurrence of treatment has an advantage in that it enables the investigator to use a class of statistical tests, simply called randomization tests, which are particularly suitable for the analysis of single-case data.

The fundamental design element in single-case experiments is the principle of frequent (repeated) measurement of the target variable that represents the clinical problem. In single-case studies, repeated measurement means many observations rather than the two, three, or four occasions of measurement that occur in RCTs. The strategy deployed in single-case designs is to establish an estimate of the individual's problem by taking repeated measures during a baseline or no-treatment phase and then to track the problem when treatment is introduced. This sequence of observations is schematized in the lower right panel of Fig. 1. When a stable baseline is observed, then if change occurs when treatment is introduced, we can be reasonably sure that the change is not attributable to factors associated with measurement or maturation issues, and provided that we can document that there were no plausible external events (history), we may conclude that the treatment is a plausible candidate as an explanation of the change. This conclusion is reinforced if we can *replicate* the experiment with other individuals using the same protocol, generating a case series.

In the terminology of single-case designs, the sequence of baseline → treatment is known as an A-B design. A refers to the baseline, and B refers to the treatment phase. In the A-B design, no attempt is made to experimentally manipulate the effect of treatment by withdrawing and then reintroducing it in an A-B-A-B sequence. The A-B-A-B design would give us greater confidence in the effectiveness of the treatment, but it is not applicable for treatments for which we expect that the treatment should produce a relatively irreversible change or where we have ethical concerns about withdrawing the treatment. As noted, we can add an element of experimental control to the A-B design by randomly allocating the point at which treatment begins. Several of case series investigating the effectiveness of graded exposure have used this strategy.

There is a range of single-case designs in which variations of the basic elements are combined to control for plausible rival hypotheses explaining the change occurring at the time of treatment [1,9,14]. In the case series reported in this chapter, we used variants on the A-B design. In one variant, we added a second treatment phase (C), graded activity, which is known to be effective from previous RCT studies. In these case series, some patients received the sequence baseline → graded exposure → graded activity (A-B-C), while others received a baseline → graded activity → graded exposure (A-C-B) sequence. We also used a second variant of the A-B design, the multiple-baseline across subjects design. In this design, participants are randomly assigned to baseline periods of different lengths before treatment. The expectation is that if treatment is responsible for change, then changes will occur only in the treatment phase. As a consequence, the graphed data will produce a staggered, step-like, response pattern across participants.

Analysis of Single-Case Studies

The evaluation of single-case data has been a point of some debate [1]. Evaluation has strongly relied on *visual analysis*, that is, interpretation of the data plot of the dependent variable over time. This method works well when there are highly stable baseline observations and rapid changes in the treatment phases, especially when experimental attempts to reverse the treatment, as in the A-B-A-B design, are present. Whatever the merits of the sole reliance on visual analysis, good data plots help both the analyst and the reader understand the data relatively easily. We will illustrate many of the studies with graphic material in Chapter 7.

Statistical analysis of single-case designs is complicated by the fact that the use of repeated measures undermines one of the fundamental assumptions of many familiar statistical tests used to detect the difference between means. Many tests assume that error terms are independent and uncorrelated; however, this cannot be taken for granted with repeated measures. There are a variety of alternative analyses; we have used both time-series analysis and randomization tests to analyze case series. We do not report the details of these here, but interested readers can refer to an excellent introduction by Onghena and Edgington [16].

Fig. 1 does not imply that RCTs do not include measurement strategies akin to single-case designs [11,18,22] or that single-case studies should not collect data at the level of standard/global measures. In our reported case-study series, we routinely asked participants to complete a range of standard/global measures. Including these measures has several advantages. First, it provides a reference point for the selection of participants. In essence, the measures can be used to calibrate the participants against available norms and to provide data to show that they are drawn from a population in which elevated scores on the measures are associated with disability and clinical need. Second, we need to demonstrate that changes produced in the study at the level of target/problem measures are reflected in changes at the construct level, as measured by standard/global measures. In our case series, we frequently set a priori criteria for improvement on standard/global measures of a 30% to 40% reduction from baseline after treatment as a marker for clinically significant change. Third, it is possible to use the psychometric characteristics of the standard/global measures to determine whether the change observed is statistically meaningful and to answer two questions: Is the change greater than can be explained by errors of measurement? And, does the endpoint (posttreatment) meet statistically defined criteria of clinical significance? [7,15].

Our case studies also used standardized measures taken pre- and posttreatment. The original publications sometimes report changes on these measures with reference to a substantial percentage change, but no statistical analyses were conducted. Normally, statistical evaluation of these measures would depend on the availability of a control group and the presence of a sufficient sample size to make meaningful comparisons. However, it is possible to conduct a more sophisticated analysis of these data for individuals than was performed in the original publications by using knowledge of the psychometric properties of the measures (reliability, standard deviation, and group norms). These properties can be used to construct answers to two important questions [6,7]. First, we can ask is the observed change at the end of treatment reliable? That is, is the change greater than the amount that could be accounted for by the fact that the measure does not possess perfect reliability? To assess this, we can use the Reliable Change Index (RCI). Classical psychometric theory recognizes that any score is not perfect but represents an estimate of the individual's true score. To assess the confidence interval for any score and to determine the magnitude of change required for that change to be regarded as *statistically* meaningful, we need two pieces of information from the test statistics: an estimate of its reliability (r) and the standard deviation (SD) of the test. The formula for estimating the standard error of measurement (SEM) is

$$\text{SEM} = \text{SD} \times \sqrt{(1 - r)},$$

and the formula for determining the reliable change index is

$$\text{RCI} = (\text{pretest score} - \text{posttest score})/\text{SE}_{\text{diff}},$$

where SE_{diff} is the standard error of the difference score and is computed as

$$\text{SE}_{\text{diff}} = \sqrt{2} \times \text{SEM}^2.$$

If the value of the RCI is greater than 1.96, we can regard the change as significant according to the traditional $P < 0.05$ criteria, that is, less than 5% chance. Note that in this formula, a decrease in the score at posttreatment is regarded as an improvement, and in this case, a positive RCI is expected.

We illustrate this approach for patients in case series 1 through 5 reported in Chapter 7 [2,10,19–21], and a summary of the analyses is shown in Table I. To compute the RCI, we need estimates of the SDs and reliability coefficients for the two tests. In this example, we selected the pooled SD from a large RCT of patients with chronic low back pain conducted in the same health care facility as case series 1 through 3 [17]. The means and SDs

Table I
Examples of Reliable Change Index and Clinical Significantly Change analyses for patients in case series 1 through 5

Case Series	Reference	Journal	Patient	RDQ				TSK			
				Pre	Post	RCI	CSC-a	Pre	Post	RCI	CSC-a
1	Vlaeyen et al. [20]	PMR	1	19	2	10.14	yes	61	22	8.98	yes
			2	16	4	7.16	yes	47	19	6.44	yes
2	Vlaeyen et al. [19]	BRAT	1	20	15	2.98	no	50	24	5.98	yes
			2*	19	4	8.94	yes	41	18	5.29	yes
			3*	12	10	*1.19*	no	41	22	4.37	yes
			4	18	12	3.58	no	50	27	5.29	no
3	Vlaeyen et al. [21]	CJP	Avg. 2	17	8	5.37	no	42	25	3.91	yes
			Avg. 3	16	3	7.75	yes	48	23	5.75	yes
4	Linton et al. [10]	CTR	1					53	44	2.07	no
			2					52	42	2.30	no
5	Boersma et al. [2]	Pain	1					54	24	6.90	yes
			2					40	30	2.30	no
			3					40	22	4.14	yes
			4								
			5					54	39	3.45	no
			6					43	20	5.29	yes

Notes: In case series 2, asterisks (*) denote that patients received graded activity before graded exposure. In case series 3, the analyses were performed on data averaged within the groups; Avg. 2 = average of two patients; Avg. 3 = average of three patients. In case series 5, patient 4 did not return data.

Measures: CSC-*a* = clinically significant change, criterion *a*; RCI = Reliable Change Index (where this figure is italicized, the change is not reliable); RDQ = Roland Disability Questionnaire; TSK = Tampa Scale of Kinesophobia.

Journal: BRAT = *Behaviour Research and Therapy*; CJP = *Clinical Journal of Pain*; CTR = *Cognitive Therapy and Research*; Pain = *Pain*; PMR = *Pain Management and Research*.

for the untreated sample were as follows: RDQ mean = 13.88, SD = 3.75; Tampa Scale for Kinesiophobia (TSK) mean = 38.83, SD = 6.87. There are various estimates of the internal reliability of both measures; we used values of 0.9 for the RDQ and 0.8 for the TSK. Table I shows the pre- and posttreatment scores for both measures followed by a column with the patient's RCI value. If this value is greater than 1.96, we can conclude that the patient made a change that is not likely to be due to an error in our measurement. Inspection shows that all but one patient made a reliable change on the RDQ, and all patients showed a reliable change on the TSK.

The second question we can answer with psychometric data is whether at the end of treatment an individual has achieved a clinically significant change. Clinical significance is a multifaceted concept, but one aspect of it can be captured statistically insofar as we regard scores above a given level (cut-point) on a test as representing dysfunction and those below the cut-point as being functional or normal. Using the cut-point, it is possible to determine whether an individual has moved from the dysfunctional to the functional range. The question then arises concerning how to define this cut-point. We could define the criterion by consensus or expert opinion; however, Jacobson and Truax [7] suggest that the statistical properties of the test be applied. Fig. 2 illustrates these properties. This figure schematizes the distribution of scores on a test from two populations, a dysfunctional population (right) and a functional one (left). In this case, they are not perfectly separated, and there is some overlap in the test scores, as is often the case with psychological variables. For an individual in the dysfunctional group, recovery is indicated by a leftward shift. Jacobson and Truax [7] suggest that three criteria based on statistical properties of the test can be used to set cut-points for clinical improvement. These are shown by the dotted vertical lines in Fig. 2. Criterion a is met when the individual moves to the extreme of the dysfunctional distribution nearest to the functional distribution. This criterion can be defined by a score in the lowest 5% of the distribution. Criterion b is met when the individual moves to within 1.96 SDs of the mean of the functional group. Criterion c is met when the individual is nearer to the functional group than to the dysfunctional group. The actual position of the points on the underlying scale will vary according to the extent to which the distributions overlap, and the choice of which criterion to use depends on the degree of overlap

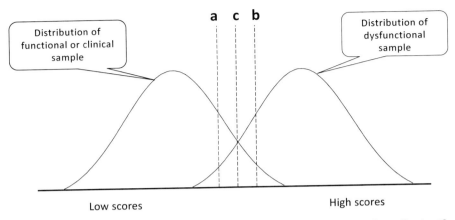

Fig. 2. Schematic representation of definitions of statistically defined clinically significant change.

between the distributions and whether data are available for a functional group. Many scales that measure dysfunction either lack data from functional groups or, where such data are available, they may have been collected from samples that are not comparable to a clinical population with regard to age and socioeconomic status. This situation often occurs when samples of convenience, often university students and employees, have been used in the development of the scales.

The results of these analyses for patients in case series is shown in Table I. For both measures, we used criterion *a*, that is, at the extreme end of the dysfunctional distribution. Using the means and SDs from the same source [17], we calculated the cut-point for the RDQ to be 6.53, and that for the TSK to be 25.36. Using these criteria, approximately half of the patients made clinically significant changes on the RDQ, and all but two made clinically significant changes on the TSK.

References

[1] Barlow DH, Nock M, Hersen M. Single case experimental designs: strategies for studying behavior change. New York: Pearson; 2009.
[2] Boersma K, Linton S, Overmeer T, Jansson M, Vlaeyen J, de Jong J. Lowering fear-avoidance and enhancing function through exposure in vivo. A multiple baseline study across six patients with back pain. Pain 2004;108:8–16.
[3] Campbell DT, Kenny D. A primer on regression artefacts. New York: Guilford; 1999.
[4] Cone JD. Evaluating outcomes empirical tools for effective practice. Washington, DC: American Psychological Association; 2000.

[5] Cook TD, Campbell DT. Quasi-experimentation: design and analysis issues for field settings. Chicago: Rand McNally; 1979.

[6] Jacobson NS, Roberts LJ, Berns SB, McGlinchey JB. Methods for defining and determining the clinical significance of treatment effects: description, application, and alternatives. J Consult Clin Psychol 1999;67:300–7.

[7] Jacobson NS, Truax P. Clinical significance: a statistical approach to defining meaningful change in psychotherapy research. J Consult Clin Psychol 1991;59:12–19.

[8] Johnson JM, Pennypacker HS. Strategies and tactics in human behavioural research. Hillsdale: Lawrence Erlbaum Associates; 1980.

[9] Kazdin AE. Single case research designs: methods for clinical and applied settings. New York: Oxford University Press; 1982.

[10] Linton SJ, Overmeer T, Janson M, Vlaeyen JWS, de Jong JR. Graded in-vivo exposure treatment for fear-avoidant pain patients with functional disability: a case study. Cogn Behav Ther 2002;31:49–58.

[11] Litt MD, Shafer DM, Ibanez CR, Kreutzer DL, Tawfik-Yonkers Z. Momentary pain and coping in temporomandibular disorder pain: exploring mechanisms of cognitive behavioral treatment for chronic pain. Pain 2009;145:160–8.

[12] McMillan D, Morley S. Single-case quantitative methods. In: Barkham M, Hardy GE, editors. A core approach to delivering practice-based evidence. Chichester: Wiley; 2010.

[13] Morley S. The dimensionality of verbal descriptors in Tursky's pain perception profile. Pain 1989;37:41–9.

[14] Morley S. Single case research. In: Parry G, Watts FN, editors. Behavioural and mental health research: a handbook of skills and methods. Hove: Lawrence Erlbaum Associates; 1996. p. 277–314.

[15] Morley S, Williams AC de C, Hussain S. Estimating the clinical effectiveness of cognitive behavioural therapy in the clinic: evaluation of a CBT informed pain management programme. Pain 2008;137:670–80.

[16] Onghena P, Edgington ES. Customization of pain treatments: single-case design and analysis. Clin J Pain 2005;21:56–68.

[17] Smeets RJ, Vlaeyen JW, Hidding A, Kester AD, van der Heijden GJ, van Geel AC, Knottnerus JA. Active rehabilitation for chronic low back pain: cognitive-behavioral, physical, or both? First direct post-treatment results from a randomized controlled trial [ISRCTN22714229]. BMC Musculoskelet Disord 2006;7:5.

[18] Turner JA, Holtzman S, Mancl L. Mediators, moderators, and predictors of therapeutic change in cognitive-behavioral therapy for chronic pain. Pain 2007;127:276–86.

[19] Vlaeyen JW, de Jong J, Geilen M, Heuts PH, van Breukelen G. Graded exposure in vivo in the treatment of pain-related fear: a replicated single-case experimental design in four patients with chronic low back pain. Behav Res Ther 2001;39:151–66.

[20] Vlaeyen JW, De Jong JR, Onghena P, Kerckhoffs-Hanssen M, Kole-Snijders AM. Can pain-related fear be reduced? The application of cognitive-behavioural exposure in vivo. Pain Res Manag 2002;7:144–53.

[21] Vlaeyen JWS, de Jong J, Geilen M, Heuts PHTG, Breukelen GV. The treatment of fear of movement/(re)injury in chronic low back pain: Further evidence on the effectiveness of exposure in vivo. Clin J Pain 2002;18:251–61.

[22] Zautra AJ, Davis MC, Reich JW, Nicassio P, Tennen H, Finan P, Kratz A, Parrish B, Irwin MR. Comparison of cognitive behavioral and mindfulness meditation interventions on adaptation to rheumatoid arthritis for patients with and without history of recurrent depression. J Consult Clin Psychol 2008;76:408–21.

Experimental Single-Case Series

In the initial test of graded exposure (GE) as a treatment, we used experimental single-case methods and have published eight articles. Each publication contains a case series, that is, more than one patient treated by the same methods, measures, and design, in what Sidman [18] and Barlow and colleagues [1] refer to as a *direct* replication. Each case series is slightly different because we examined variations in specific hypotheses tested and generalized the basic observations to new settings, therapists, and disorders. The set of studies therefore constitutes a *systematic* replication of the treatment. A summary of the eight articles is shown in Table I.

Notwithstanding the variations across the studies, we maintained a common approach to measurement that captured data at both the standard/global level and the target level. In each case series, we obtained measures before baseline observations and after each phase of treatment, as well as at follow-up time points. We also kept two measures of fear of movement/(re)injury constant in all studies (i.e., the Tampa Scale for Kinesiophobia [TSK] and the Photograph Series of Daily Activities [PHODA]). In addition, we used the well-known Roland-Morris Disability Questionnaire (RDQ) to measure functional disability in patients with back pain. This instrument was replaced by more specific measures for studies of patients with neck pain and complex regional pain syndrome type I (CRPS-I).

Pain-Related Fear: Exposure-Based Treatment for Chronic Pain
by Johan W.S. Vlaeyen, Stephen J. Morley, Steven J. Linton, Katja Boersma, and Jeroen de Jong
IASP Press, Seattle, © 2012

Table I
Summary of single-case studies of graded exposure treatment

Study	Authors	Journal [Ref.]	Year	Purpose	Group	N	Design	Measure TSK	PHODA	RDQ	Other
1	Vlaeyen et al.	PRM [22]	2002	To establish validity	CLBP	2	AB	Y	Y	Y	
2	Vlaeyen et al.	BRAT [21]	2001	To compare with alternative treatment of graded activity	CLBP	4	ABC	Y	Y	Y	PVAQ, PCL
3	Vlaeyen et al.	CJP [23]	2002	To add "direct" measure of activity	CLBP	6	ABC	Y	Y	Y	
4	Linton et al.	CBT [10]	2002	To test viability in other setting (country)	CLBP	2	Pre/post	Y	Y	Y	
5	Boersma et al.	Pain [2]	2004	Replication by other therapists, with other setting and design	CLBP	6	Multiple baseline across subjects	N	Y	N	Örebro scales
6	de Jong et al.	CJP [5]	2005	To test effect of education component of graded exposure	CLBP	8	ABC/D	Y	Y	Y	
7	de Jong et al.	Pain [4]	2005	To test validity for a non-musculoskeletal disorder	CRPS-1	8	ABC	Y	Y		QRS, WSQ, RASQ
8	de Jong et al.	J Pain [3]	2008	To test validity for other musculoskeletal disorder	Whip-lash	8	ABC	Y	Y	Y	NDI

Journal: BRAT = *Behaviour Research and Therapy;* CBT = *Cognitive Behaviour Therapy;* CJP = *Clinical Journal of Pain;* J Pain = *Journal of Pain;* Pain = *Pain;* PRM = *Pain Research and Management. Group:* CLBP = chronic low back pain; CRPS-1 = complex regional pain syndrome, type I; whiplash = neck pain arising from a whiplash event in a motor vehicle accident. *N* = number of individuals in the study. *Design:* A = baseline; B = treatment, graded exposure; C = treatment or comparator treatment (D), e.g., graded activity. *Measures:* NDI = Neck Disability Questionnaire; PCL = Pain Cognition List; PHODA = Photograph Series of Daily Activities; PVAQ = Pain Vigilance and Awareness Questionnaire; QRS = Questionnaire on Rising and Sitting; RASQ = Radboud Skills Questionnaire; RDQ = Roland Disability Questionnaire; TSK = Tampa Scale for Kinesiophobia; WSQ = Walking Stairs Questionnaire. All references for the measures are given in the text.

Single-case designs require that measures of the therapeutic target are taken at frequent and regular intervals. In the studies that follow, we have for the most part used a daily dairy completed by the patients. The core of this diary (11 items) is shown in Table II. The diary comprises items taken from standard scales to measure beliefs and appraisals central to the cognitive-behavioral fear-avoidance model, which include fear of movement/(re)injury (TSK, four items); fear of pain (Pain Anxiety Symptoms Scale [PASS], four items); and catastrophizing (Pain Catastrophizing Scale [PCS], three items). Each of these items was presented in the diary, and patients were asked to rate them on a 10-cm visual analogue scale (VAS) anchored by the phrases "totally agree" and "totally disagree." We also included a single VAS to measure daily pain intensity anchored by the phrases "no pain at all" and "worst pain experienced." In several studies, we also included items selected by the individual that reflected key behavioral activities in which they wished to re-engage. More details on these items are included with each case series.

Table II

Items of the shortened and adapted versions of the Tampa Scale for Kinesiophobia (TSK), Pain Anxiety Symptoms Scale (PASS), and Pain Catastrophizing Scale (PCS) selected for the daily diary used in case studies 1–3 and 6–8

TSK: Fear of Movement/(Re)injury

1) If I exercise, I might be in danger of reinjuring myself. (Harm)
2) My body is telling me I have something dangerously wrong. (Fear)
3) My pain complaints would decrease if I were to exercise. (Exercise)
4) I can't do everything because it's too easy for me to get injured. (Avoidance)

PASS: Anxiety about Pain

1) I become sweaty when in pain. (Somatic anxiety)
2) I feel confused when I hurt. (Cognitive anxiety)
3) When I feel pain, I think that something dreadful may happen. (Fear)
4) When I feel pain, I try to stay as still as possible. (Escape/avoidance)

PCS: Catastrophizing

1) When I am in pain, I keep thinking about how badly I want the pain to stop. (Rumination)
2) When I am in pain, I wonder whether something serious may happen. (Magnification)
3) When I am in pain, I feel I can't go on with my daily activities. (Helplessness)

Note: The subscales from which the items are drawn are shown in parentheses. Each item was accompanied by a 10-cm visual analog scale anchored by the phrases "totally disagree" and "totally agree" and scored to the nearest millimeter.

Case Series 1: Can Pain-Related Fear Be Reduced by Behavioral In Vivo Exposure?

The first case series [22] simply aimed to determine whether pain-related fear can be reduced using the method of GE. The case series used the basic A-B design with two female patients ages 45 and 47 years who had had back pain for 1 and 12 years, respectively. Each patient kept the standard diary for 42 days, and the data from these diaries was used to track their progress. Both patients started with a 1-week baseline period (no treatment) followed by 15 treatment sessions of 90 minutes each over a 5-week period. No other treatment was given during this time. We also obtained data with the TSK, PHODA, and RDQ before and after treatment. Data for both patients' daily ratings of fear of movement and pain intensity are plotted in Fig. 1. Inspection of these plots shows that both patients had a reasonably stable baseline on the two measures and that within a few days of the start of treatment, their daily ratings of fear of movement dropped quite dramatically to the minimum. It is also evident that both patients recorded a large drop in their ratings of pain. In one case, this resulted in an almost complete reduction of pain, whereas in the other, it was consistently reduced from ~8 to ~3 on the 10-cm VAS scale.

This visual analysis of the data was supported by randomization tests of the two data sets. Under the assumption that treatment could have been randomized to start with a minimum of 5 days baseline up to a maximum of 37 days of treatment, there are 33 possible combinations

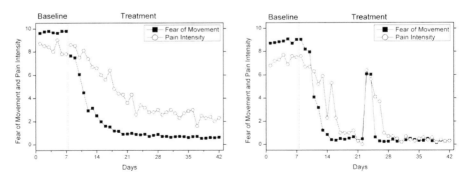

Fig. 1. Daily measures of fear and pain intensity for the two patients treated in case series 1 [22].

of baseline and treatment duration, giving a possible minimum value of $P = 0.0303$. Analyses for both patients indicated that significant changes in fear of movement were attained within 1 to 3 days after the start of treatment, and pain intensity was significantly reduced by days 4 and 5 post-treatment. Randomization tests were also conducted on pain catastrophizing and fear of pain, and both of these measures showed a significant reduction within 2 to 4 days after the start of treatment. The patients also showed marked reductions on all of the standard global measures: TSK, PHODA, RDQ, and the Pain Vigilance and Awareness Questionnaire (PVAQ) (see Table 5 in the original publication).

This initial case series provided some evidence that GE might be a viable treatment for patients with high levels of fear of pain-related movement, but the relatively short baseline, no plausible control treatment, and only two patients severely limited the degree of confidence in the generality of the results.

Case Series 2: Replication and Extension

The second case series [21] was conducted with four patients, three women and one man aged 31 to 40 years, with chronic low back pain. These patients (patients 1-4) had had pain for 5 to 20 years and showed marked disabilities, with RDQ scores ranging from 15 to 18 at the start of the case series. In this case series, two alterations were made to the simple A-B design of case series 1. First, the baseline period of no treatment was extended to 3 weeks. This extension had the advantage of allowing us to determine the stability of the measures, and it also allowed for a parametric time-series statistical analysis of the data. The second alteration was the addition a comparator treatment condition, graded activity (GA), to the design. Graded activity is based on the operant conditioning method first described by Fordyce [6], in which activity quotas are developed with the agreement of the patient. The patient is asked to follow the quota on a time-contingent schedule. In practice, an exercise circuit with various items of fitness equipment is provided, and individual exercises are selected on the basis of observations during the baseline period and the observed physical work demands. In the present case series, there was one restriction; to avoid contamination with graded-exposure treatment, any activities placed above 50 on the PHODA fear-thermometer were excluded. This rule was monitored by the physical therapist, and the patient was not aware of it. The design of the case series was also altered to incorporate the addition of the GA. All patients started with the 3-week baseline, and thereafter, two were randomized to either 3 weeks of graded in vivo exposure (GE) followed by 3 weeks of GA (patients 1 and 4) or the alternate sequence (patients 2 and 3). In the terminology of single-case design, the two sequences were A-B-C or A-C-B. The interventions were delivered by an experienced team who provided a comprehensive rehabilitation service in an inpatient setting.

Time-series data for the three separate measures contained in the diary (pain-related fear, fear of pain-related movement, and catastrophizing) from two patients (patients 2 and 4 in the original publication) who received the interventions in different order are shown in Fig. 2. Patient 2 received GA before GE (left column). Inspection shows a relatively stable baseline for all measures followed by little change when the GA program was introduced and a marked reduction for all three measures within 2 to 5 days after the start of GE. This pattern was replicated for patient 3 (not shown in Fig. 2), who received the same sequence of treatments as patient 2. The right column of Fig. 2 shows the data for patient 4. After the 3-week, no-treatment baseline, she received GE, and again the data show a marked reduction in her beliefs regarding fear, activity and catastrophizing. After treatment, the levels for all three measures were almost at the minimum possible level, and it is not surprising that no further reduction could be observed in the GA treatment phase. This pattern was also shown for patient 1, who received the same sequence of treatments as patient 4. Statistical analysis of the data by autoregressive time-series modeling confirmed the impressions given by visual inspection of the data, that changes in the key measures of belief and catastrophizing occurred with GE treatment, and little change occurred with GA treatment.

A plot of scores on the three standardized measures (TSK, PHODA, RDQ) for patients 2 and 4 at four key points in the experiment, baseline, before the first treatment (either GA or GE), after the first treatment, and after the second treatment, is shown in Fig. 3. The shaded bar indicates the occurrence of the graded-exposure treatment. Inspection of the plot shows that the marked reduction in all three measures occurred after

GE treatment, but little change occurred after GA treatment. The same pattern was replicated for patients 1 and 3 (data not shown).

The data from this case series not only replicated the effect of graded-exposure treatment but also indicated that the effect was due to some specific component in the treatment rather than simply the presence of an active, well-structured, and competently delivered treatment such as GA. As Vlaeyen and colleagues noted ([21] p. 162), "Exposure was not the sole treatment provided to these patients, but was embedded in a comprehensive rehabilitation program that followed an operant treatment regimen, provided by the whole multidisciplinary treatment staff. However, the GE and GA were principally given by the physical therapist and the health scientist. Although the supplemental value of this 'background' treatment program cannot be ruled out in this case series, the remarkable improvements that are observed whenever the graded exposure was initiated suggests that the therapeutic power of the graded exposure is much

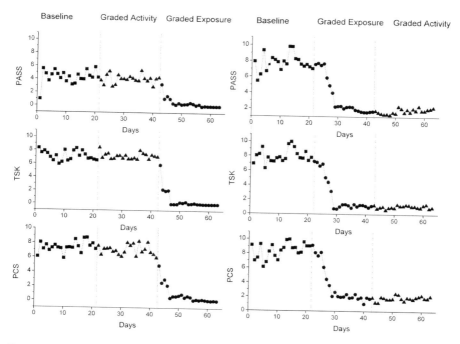

Fig. 2. Daily diary measures of items assessing pain anxiety (PASS), fear of movement (TSK), and catastrophizing (PCS) for patients 2 (left side) and 4 (right side) from study [21] in case series 2. A = baseline (■), B = graded exposure (●), C = graded activity (▲).

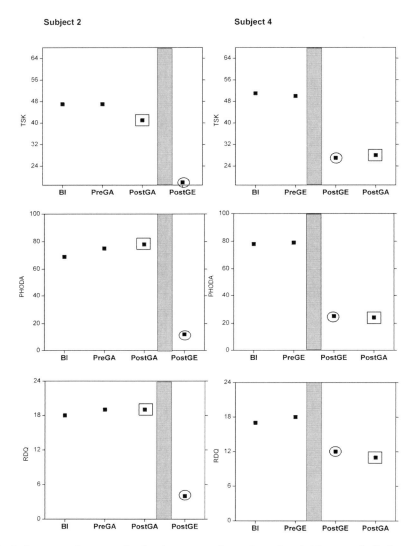

Fig. 3. Scores on three standardized measures for patients 2 and 4 from study [21] in case series 2. Bl = baseline; PreGA = before graded activity; PostGA = after graded activity (□); PreGE = before graded exposure, PostGE = after graded exposure (○). The shaded bar indicates the transition between the graded exposure and graded activity treatments.

stronger. The crossover design gave us the opportunity to examine the differential effects of graded exposure and graded activity and the additional treatment effect of the second therapy module. As the order of treatment modules did not make any difference on the final outcome, no such effect was found in this case series. On the other hand, (desirable) carry-over effects were clearly observed when graded exposure was followed by graded activity."

Although results of this case series replicated those of case series 1, it was based on relatively few patients ($n = 4$). One authority on single-case design suggests a rule of thumb for the minimum number of cases as one successful case and three replications [1]. Case series 2 just meets this minimum criterion; however, an exacting critic might point out that because there were only two patients in each treatment sequence, we might wish to be more circumspect about any claim of robust replication.

Case Series 3: Further Evidence of the Effectiveness of Graded Exposure

Case series 3 [23] was designed as a direct replication of case series 2, using the same design to contrast the relative effect of GE and GA treatments with the same core set of measures. The length of the three phases (A, Baseline; B, GE; C, GA) was extended to 4 weeks, and two additional features were added. First, we attempted to add a direct measure of physical activity. The fear-avoidance model is explicit in its prediction that a reduction in fear appraisals should be accompanied by an increase in behavioral activity, with an associated reduction in disability. Case series 1 and 2 obtained indirect data on behavior and disability using the RDQ. In case series 3, this information was supplemented with the use of an ambulatory activity monitor (uniaxial accelerometer) attached to a belt close to lumbar disks L4 and L5. The accelerometer recorded movements, except for activities involving contact with water such as taking a shower or swimming, during the patient's waking hours for an entire week. Patients kept track of the time when they carried the accelerometer and the kind of activities they performed in a diary. The activity monitor was carried three times for an entire week for the baseline, GE treatment, and GA treatment phases.

The second change to the protocol was made because we were concerned that differences between the efficacy of GE and GA treatments might be attributable to differences in the perceived credibility of the treatments and patients' expectations of outcomes that could be achieved. We therefore asked patients three questions about the perceived credibility of the treatment and their expectations of outcomes at the end of each of the first treatment sessions, as follows:

1) Do you expect that the program will help you to cope better with your pain complaints?
2) Do you expect that the program will help patients with chronic back pain in general cope better with their pain complaints?
3) Do you believe that the treatment offered to you is a meaningful treatment for patients with back pain?

Patients rated each item on a VAS, with "not at all" and "very much" as the anchors, and a credibility score was calculated as the mean for the three items (possible maximum, 10). The mean ratings for both treatments were high, at 8.7 and 8.6 for GE and GA, respectively.

Nine consecutive patients with chronic low back pain were assessed. Two were excluded because they did not meet the inclusion criteria, and one patient discontinued treatment after 3 weeks because of a deterioration in marital and family circumstances. The remaining 4 female and 2 male patients completed the case series. Their ages ranged from 26 to 51 years, and they had had pain for 3 to 7 years. Two patients had had prior surgery. Three patients were randomized to each treatment sequence.

Composite data (averaged for the three patients in each treatment sequence) for the daily diary ratings of fear of movement/(re)injury plotted across the 12 weeks of the case series are shown in Fig. 4. The lower panel shows data for patients who received GE before GA. Following the relatively stable baseline, there was a marked reduction in levels of reported fear of movement with the introduction of graded-exposure treatment, to the point where reported levels of fear were minimal. Not surprisingly, there was no additional improvement with the introduction of GA treatment. Individual data plots resembled the averaged data, and similar patterns were observed for the measures of catastrophizing and fear of pain.

By way of contrast, the upper panel of Fig. 4 in shows that when GA was the first treatment, there was little change in reports of fear of movement and that this only changed when GE treatment was introduced. As with the other treatment group, the averaged data plot was mirrored by the individual data plots. Statistical analysis with the same

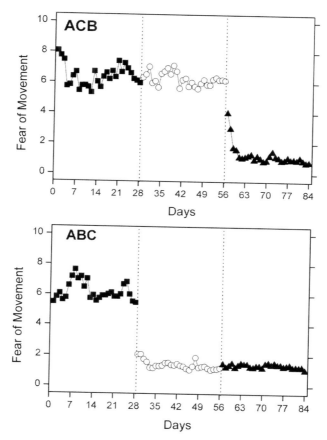

Fig. 4. Composite daily diary data for fear of movement (TSK) for the two treatment sequences in case series 3 [23]. A = baseline (■), B = graded exposure (○), C = graded activity (▲).

autoregressive modeling techniques used in case series 2 confirmed that statistically significant changes in fear of movement/(re)injury, fear of pain, and catastrophizing occurred with the introduction of GE treatment but not after GA treatment. There was also a reduction in pain intensity reported after GE treatment.

The standardized measures (TSK, RDQ, and PCS) also showed the same pattern of change, with marked reductions following the introduction of GE treatment but not with GA treatment (see Table 4 in [23]). To analyze the activity data, the statistical distribution of each patient's baseline data, calculated as the deviation of the mean activity levels in the GE and GA treatment phases from the baseline, was expressed as a z-score (a z-score of greater than +1.96 indicated that the average activity in the treatment phase was at the 97.5 percentile of baseline activity). The z-scores for the patients receiving the A-B-C sequence were 4.84, 2.96, and 14.86 after B (GE) and 4.26, 2.83, and 15.44 after C (GA), indicating that behavioral activity increased significantly after treatment with GE and was maintained after GA. The z-scores for the group treated in the reverse sequence, A-C-B, were: 1.76, 0.44, and 2.37 after C (GA) and 3.70, 2.33, and 12.24 after B (GE), indicating that only one patient significantly increased behavioral activity after GA but that all patients increased their behavioral activity after GE.

In summary, this case series successfully replicated case series 2 and provided preliminary evidence that differences between the two treatments' effectiveness do not appear to be attributable to differences in their perceived credibility or expectation of treatment gain and that behavioral activity increased after GE treatment.

Case Series 4 and 5: Generalizing the Observations to Another Health System and Country

Case series 1 through 3 were carried out by a clinical research team in The Netherlands. The next two series [2,10] provide evidence for the generalization of the methods to a different country, Sweden, with a different health care system and different therapists. There is an extensive history of liaison between the two research groups, and the Maastricht group provided training and supervision for the group based in Örebro. In the Swedish group's first case series, case series 4 [10], an attempt was made to replicate the treatment for two patients with low back pain. The therapy team, comprising two physical therapists and a clinical psychologist, conducted the case series in a primary care setting with two male patients, a 54-year-old with a history of low back pain since adolescence and a 57-year-old with a 3-year history of back pain after a motor-vehicle accident. The entry criteria for this case series were (1) absence of any indicators of serious physical pathology, for example, cauda equina syndrome,

(2) a score of 24 or greater on the three items of fear-avoidance from the Örebro Musculoskeletal Pain Screening Questionnaire [9], and (3) a willingness to participate. The PHODA, TSK, and daily diary were also translated into Swedish for use in this case series. Whereas the PHODA and TSK were used successfully, the two participants found the diary difficult to use and complained that the items were not clear. There were many missing data values, and the diary was discontinued. Therefore, it was not possible to complete the case series as intended in the form of an A-B time-series design.

Patients were seen for one education session and eight 40-minute treatment sessions during a 5-week period. Data were available for the standard measures PHODA and TSK, and simple pre- to post-treatment comparisons were made. Both patients showed very modest reductions in their TSK scores (Patient 1, 53 to 44; Patient 2, 52 to 44). Whereas both of these changes represent a statistically reliable change the post-treatment scores were greater than the mean (39) for the TSK. Similar modest changes were noted in the PHODA scores (Patient 1, 71 to 51; Patient 2, 62 to 47). Despite these modest gains in the standardized measures, both patients completed the treatment hierarchies, reported little fear or worry about the activities at the end of treatment, and began to engage in activities at home that they had previously avoided such as cutting wood.

The relative success of this pilot case series led to the development of a second case series [2] with six patients. Adaptations of the daily diary were made to improve its usability for the Swedish population. A five-item diary was developed to assess fear and avoidance beliefs and pain, selecting specific items from published questionnaires and writing items when necessary. The final diary items and their origins are as follows:

1) Physical activity makes my pain worse. (Fear Avoidance Beliefs Questionnaire [FABQ] [25])
2) To what degree are you worried that physical activity can worsen your pain? (Designed for the case series)
3) How worried are you about your back problem? (From [24])
4) An increase in pain is an indication that I should stop what I am doing until the pain decreases. (Pain and Impairment Relationship Scale [PAIRS] [13])
5) How much pain do you have today? (Designed for the case series)

All items were scored on a 0-to-10 scale. Other measures included another questionnaire especially constructed from several sources and administered weekly to assess function and fear and avoidance beliefs (five items for each component). The TSK and PHODA were used as standard measures. A screening questionnaire was constructed from items drawn from PAIRS [13], the Örebro Musculoskeletal Pain Screening Questionnaire [9], FABQ [25], and items from the back pain worry questions of Von Korff and colleagues [24].

Whereas participants in the Maastricht studies were recruited from a tertiary-level rehabilitation clinic, the Örebro case series recruited participants from the general population via an advertisement in a local newspaper. A total of 80 individuals were screened by telephone. Inclusion criteria were (1) age 18 to 60 years, (2) duration of back pain of at least 6 months, (3) problems with functioning, and (4) absence of indicators of a serious physical condition related to back pain. A physician screened the individuals before final acceptance into the case series. A total of 46 individuals fulfilled the criteria and were further screened with the TSK, PHODA, and the fear and avoidance screening measure constructed for the case series. Cut-off scores for inclusion in the case series were greater than 35 on the TSK (range 17–68) and greater than 60 on the fear and avoidance measure (range 0–90). In addition, at least 30 of the 98 items of the PHODA had to be rated at greater than 50, and at least 15 of those had to be rated greater than 80. Twelve individuals fulfilled these criteria, and the six with the highest scores on the measures were invited to participate. The subjects were ages 34 to 61 years and had experienced pain for 3 to 20 years.

In case series 5 [2], the single-case design was also changed to a between-subjects, multiple baseline design. Each subject recorded daily diary ratings during a baseline period (no treatment), a treatment period, and a subsequent follow-up period (no treatment). The total duration of the case series for each subject was 10 weeks. The critical experimental variable between subjects was the duration of the baseline period. For one subject, this period was relatively short (1 week), but it increased by 1 week for each of the other subjects, such that the last subject recorded baseline data for 6 weeks. Treatment was introduced for subjects at the end of their allocated baseline period. The logic underlying the multiple baseline design is that if the treatment is responsible for change, the change will occur only at the point of intervention. When the data are plotted, the resulting graph will appear as a step-like sequence as the baseline period extends. If alternative mechanisms of change, for example, maturation, history, or statistical regression to the mean, are responsible for the change, we would have to believe that these coincided exactly with the period in which the treatment was introduced. This coincidence becomes less and less plausible as the number of subjects and baseline period increases (for a more detailed and critical discussion of the logic of this design, see [1,8,11]).

The daily diary data are shown in Fig. 5. Inspection of the data suggests that for subjects 1, 3, 4, and 6 the introduction of treatment was followed by a reduction in the daily diary ratings of fear and avoidance, although the rate at which the reduction occurred was not as fast as that seen in earlier studies. Subject 2 appears to have made a slow improvement during the study period, and the data also suggest that this reduction in

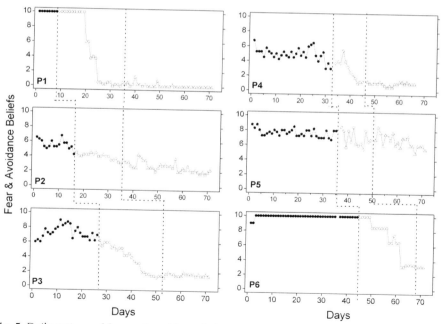

Fig. 5. Daily ratings of fear and avoidance beliefs for six patients in the multiple baseline case series 5 [2]. The figure has been redrawn from the original dataset. Baseline = ■, graded exposure = □, follow-up = Δ. The dotted lines show the beginning and end of the active treatment periods.

fear and avoidance was occurring during the baseline period. We should therefore exercise great caution in attributing the change for this subject to the introduction of GE. Similarly, subject 5 appears to have experienced a reduction in reported fear and avoidance, but it was slight compared to the other subjects.

Changes observed in the daily diary data were reflected in TSK scores taken pre- and post-treatment and at the 3-month follow-up (with the exception of patient 4, who did not provide data). For patients 1, 3, and 6 there were marked reductions in TSK scores from greater than 40 to ~20. These improvements were sustained at follow-up. Such changes were not observed in patients 2 and 5. Data obtained on the PHODA for patients 1 to 3, 5, and 6 showed similar improvements (reductions in fear) from baseline to treatment and follow-up. It will be recalled that this case series used a nonstandard measure of function, and so the interpretation and analysis of this measure is more problematic. Nevertheless, the scores on this measure did change markedly in the direction of improvement (see Table 5 in the original publication).

Results of these two studies provide preliminary evidence that graded-exposure treatment might be effective beyond the confines of its place of development. Case series 5 replicated the findings of case series 1 through 3 in a new setting, with new therapists, using a different experimental design and with some of the measures developed for that setting. Compared to the 12 patients treated in case series 1 through 3, the magnitude of improvement for the patients in case series 4 and 5 was not as uniformly substantial. The reasons for this are not clear. The experience of the team in Örebro was obviously limited compared to that of the original group in Maastricht. Boersma and colleagues [2] observed that the therapists in the Swedish team noted that they required new "skills to deal with the intricacies of exposure, especially discovering the most fear provoking activities and addressing inappropriate beliefs." There was also one other significant difference in this case series in that the patients received only the exposure treatment, whereas patients in the Dutch facility experienced exposure embedded within a comprehensive rehabilitation program. Nevertheless, the results of this case series were encouraging and suggest that the treatment can be generalized to other locations.

Case Series 6: Education or Exposure?

Although compared to many cognitive-behavioral treatments for chronic pain, graded in vivo exposure is a simple treatment insofar as it does not have multiple treatment components, there is a substantial education component at the beginning of the treatment. In the next case series [5], we sought to investigate the potential role of the education component in producing changes in beliefs and behavior. Recall that the act of GE is always preceded by careful assessment and formulation (case conceptualization), during which the fear-avoidance model is presented to patients in a personalized format explicitly linking their particular beliefs and behavior. In essence, the model is used to provide a highly personalized account to the patient and it provides a detailed rationale for the ensuing treatment. In case series 1 through 5, this component was provided during the first treatment session. In theory, it is possible that the individualized education session might be responsible for change in behavior. In case series 6, we used two treatment sequences applied to two groups of three patients each. In the first sequence, A-B-C, the baseline (A) was followed by a single education session, after which there was a period of 21 days of no intervention. We anticipated that this period would be sufficient for the single education session to take effect and for patients to initiate their own behavioral change if education were effective in its own right. Following this period, graded in vivo exposure was delivered for a 6-week period. In the A-B-D treatment sequence, the operant GA program used in previous studies followed the education session.

Patients kept daily records of their fear appraisals, beliefs, and pain using the diary as in earlier case series. In this case series, we introduced an additional component to the daily diary by asking patients to nominate three personally relevant activities. The difficulty in performing these activities was rated with a 10-cm VAS scale anchored with "no problem at all" and "impossible." The standardized measures—PHODA, TSK, RDQ, and PVAQ [14]—were administered before and after the education and treatment phases and at a 6-month follow-up. An ambulatory activity monitor was used to record activity for 1 week in each phase of the case series (baseline, education, treatment, and follow-up).

Fig. 6, in which the data have been aggregated across patients, shows that in each treatment sequence the education intervention produced a decrease in the daily measures of fear, catastrophizing, and beliefs about movement-related harm. Statistical analysis using randomization tests supported this interpretation in that for both treatment sequences there were statistically significant reductions in the daily diary measures. The data marked with an open square in Fig. 6 show the results for the three patients who received the graded-exposure treatment after the education session. The data plot indicates a further reduction in the daily measure of fear-related beliefs that was maintained at follow-up. This interpretation was also supported by the pattern of statistically significant change. The data marked with an open circle show the results of the three patients who received the GA program after the education

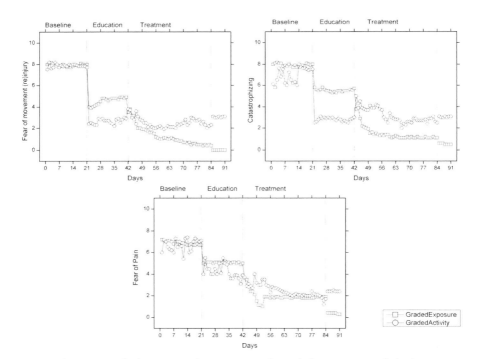

Fig. 6. The impact of education and treatment with graded exposure on daily diary measures fear of movement, catastrophizing, and fear of pain in case series 6. The data have been aggregated across individuals for two treatment sequences: ABC (baseline, education, graded exposure (□) and ABD (baseline, education, operant [graded activity]) (o). The final seven data points are from follow-up at 6 months. Redrawn from [5, Fig. 1].

session. Here, the pattern suggested that no additional changes occurred when GA was introduced and that at follow-up there appeared to be a slight deterioration, although this did not appear to be very great. Indeed, the randomization test analysis confirmed the visual analysis in that for this group, no further significant gains were made during the GA period.

Plots of the daily diary reports of difficulty engaging in behavioral activity are shown in Fig. 7 for two patients. There was a subtle difference between the patterns observed in these data from those seen in the daily record of beliefs. This was particularly so for the group treated with GE. In these three patients, very little change in self-reported behavioral performance occurred during the education phase. This interpretation is supported by data from the activity monitor, which showed no change in activity during the education phase. In contrast, all three patients showed very substantial reductions in difficulty in performing behavioral tasks when GE was introduced. This finding was supported by similar substantial increases in activity recorded on the activity monitor, with an average z score of approximately +30. Behavioral performance in the three patients receiving the education–graded-exposure sequence was more variable. Patient 2 showed some improvement after the education phase, but this did not appear to be sustained when GA was introduced. The other two patients receiving this sequence of treatment made modest gains in their behavioral performance, but the gains did not appear to be consistently related to either treatment phase. Analysis of activity monitor data showed little change during the education phase and, compared to the graded-exposure group, a modest increase with the introduction of GA.

Results of this case series provided additional evidence for the efficacy of GE as a treatment. Specifically, the results suggest that the highly individualized provision of information based on extensive data collection and systematized by the fear-avoidance model reduces self-reported pain-related fear appraisals (fear and catastrophizing) and that these changes were sustained for a period of 3 weeks after the single intervention session. However, this intervention was not sufficient to induce substantial behavioral changes, which did, however, occur when GE was introduced, but not when GA was introduced.

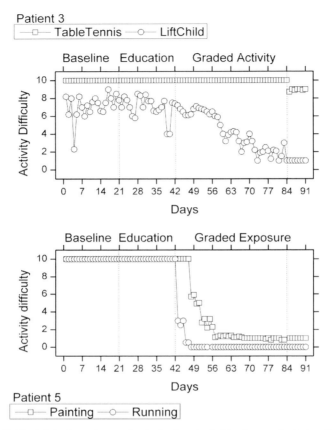

Fig. 7. Individual data from two patients for two individually nominated activities in case series 6. Patient 3 received the graded activity treatment, and patient 5 received graded exposure. The visual analogue scale records the daily difficulty in engaging in the activity (10 = "impossible," 0 = "no problem at all"). Redrawn from [5, Fig. 2].

Case Series 7 and 8: Generalizing the Treatment to Neck Pain and CRPS-I

The final two case series demonstrate that the fear-avoidance model can be generalized beyond chronic low back pain to two other diagnostic groups. One group is another musculoskeletal disorder, neck pain attributable to a "whiplash" injury [3], and the other comprises patients with CRPS-I, which has been difficult to treat with psychological methods [4].

The first of these studies [4] applied the principles of fear avoidance to eight female patients (mean age, 40 years) with diagnosed CRPS-I.

Two had pain in the lower right extremity, one had pain in the lower left extremity, one had pain in the upper left extremity, and four had pain in the upper right extremity. At first thought, the applicability of the fear-avoidance model to this group might appear rather surprising; however, we conjectured that hyperalgesia and allodynic sensitivity to pain could lead to excessive guarding and overprotective behavior, which we construe as avoidance behavior that can lead to disability. In support of this, there was evidence of elevated TSK scores in this group.

Case series 7 was also designed to separate the education and treatment phases of treatment as in case series 6. There were four phases, a baseline period (A) followed by a single education session (B), in which the patient was presented with a highly personalized formulation of the problem along with the rationale for treatment. At this point, the perceived credibility of the pending treatment and the expectation that it would help them cope better with the pain complaint were assessed. After the education session, the treatment phase (GE) was started. This phase lasted for 10 weeks, consisting of two treatment sessions per week, 1 hour each. Finally, there was a single week of data recording at the 6-month follow-up. To provide some experimental control, the baseline and education phases were varied at 7 days or 14 days in a two-by-two between-subjects design. The patients were randomly assigned to one of the four possible combinations. This simple variation provided some protection against the threats to validity posed by maturation and history.

As in the earlier case series, we used a daily diary to record fear of movement, pain anxiety, catastrophizing, pain intensity and two additional items, in which patients rated their difficulty in performing personally relevant activities. The standardized measures included the TSK and PHODA; however, the RDQ was replaced by measures of disability with greater relevance for this patient group. For patients with upper extremity pain, we used the Radboud Skills Questionnaire [12]. For those with lower limb pain, we used the Walking Stairs Questionnaire (WSQ) [17] and the Questionnaire on Rising and Sitting (QRS) [15,16].

The extension of GE to CRPS-I appears an unlikely step, and this skepticism was reflected in the patients' ratings of the credibility of the treatment and expectation of gain obtained after the education session. In contrast to data obtained in the previous case series, these patients were skeptical about the treatment (credibility mean = 4.2 ± 0.79) and rated the expectation of gain as only 3.4 (±0.84) on the 10-cm VAS scale. Despite this initial skepticism, the treatment appeared to be effective, although the pattern of change was subtly different from that in the earlier studies of musculoskeletal pain.

Data from two patients illustrating the findings of this case series are shown in Fig. 8 (data for all patients are shown in the original publication). There were a number of features in these plots. First, during the

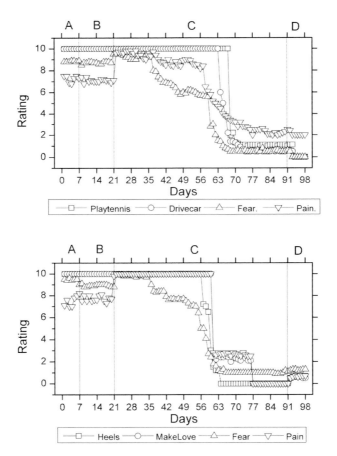

Fig. 8. Daily diary data for two patients in case series 7, showing ratings of the ease with which they could carry out two individually nominated activities: playing tennis and driving a car; wearing high-heeled shoes and making love. Patients also rated their fear of movement and pain. The experimental phases were: A = baseline, B = education session, C = graded exposure, D = follow-up. Redrawn from [4, Fig. 4].

baseline phase, patients reported very high levels of pain, fear of movement, and difficulty in performing their chosen tasks. Second, and unlike the previous data for patients with musculoskeletal pain, there was no evidence that the personalized formulation and education session had any effect at all on their ratings. Third, there was no immediate reduction in any of the key variables when treatment was introduced. However, treatment gains were consistently observed between 3 and 4 weeks after the onset of treatment, that is, after 6 to 8 treatment sessions. When change occurred, there appeared to be an initial reduction in fear of movement, after which both the level of pain experienced and the difficulty in performing selected activities decreased substantially. Randomization tests confirmed the lagged intervention effect for most patients, with significant reductions in pain intensity and fear of movement occurring by the sixth week of treatment. Although Fig. 8 (and the original article's figures) suggested that fear of movement and pain intensity showed reductions before changes in behavioral performance, statistical tests could not confirm this because of the way the lag was defined for the purpose of analysis. A fourth notable feature was that the onset of treatment was nearly always accompanied by a significant increase in the patient's level of pain. In the data shown in Fig. 8, patients' daily pain intensity abruptly increased from ~7 to almost maximum (10) for a period of 1 or 2 weeks at the onset of treatment.

Analyses of the standard measures showed that the TSK (mean = 54.75, standard deviation [SD] = 5.18) was unaffected by the education phase (mean = 55.0, SD = 5.24); however, it dropped to almost the minimum possible value (17) post-treatment (mean = 20.85, SD = 3.05) and at follow-up (mean = 19.75, SD = 1.67). This reduction was equivalent to moving from the 80th to the 10th percentile on the TSK scale. The PHODA data showed a similar pattern, with no change attributable to the education phase (baseline mean = 84.75, SD = 3.96; education mean = 85.5, SD = 3.82) but a large reduction at the end of treatment (mean = 12.86, SD = 3.31), which was maintained at follow-up (mean = 11.63, SD = 2.33). The various specific measures of functional disability also showed significant decrements in all domains (see Tables 2 and 3 in the original publication). Also of note was that virtually all of the patients showed complete loss of the clinical signs and symptoms by follow-up. No patient had hyperalgesia, edema, skin color or temperature asymmetry, or changes in sweating.

There are several notable differences between the results observed in case series 7 and earlier series. Given the lag between the start of treatment and the onset of treatment response, can we be sure that the gains were attributable to treatment? As noted earlier, the plausibility of interpreting a treatment effect in single-case designs is enhanced if gains occur shortly after treatment onset; however, the present pattern of results went against that. Alternative explanations, such as maturation, history, and measurement artifacts, might be considered; however, we suggest that these explanations are implausible. The reason for this stance is that despite the delay in the onset of response, the pattern was remarkably consistent in that it occurred during the sixth week of treatment in all eight cases. It appears implausible that history, measurement, or maturation threats would have occurred with such remarkable consistency. We therefore tentatively concluded that the changes were attributable to GE, although the exact mechanism underlying the delay in treatment response has yet to be determined. One other difference between this case series and the earlier ones is notable. All of the patients with CRPS-I showed marked reductions in pain intensity as part of the treatment response. This response has not always been observed in patients with musculoskeletal pain, for whom reductions in pain have been less marked and more variable.

The final case series (case series 8) [3] investigated the effectiveness of GE in the treatment of musculoskeletal pain arising from post-traumatic neck pain after a whiplash-related injury. The case series design, A-B-C, emulated the one used for case series 2. Eight patients who had had neck pain for longer than 12 weeks after a road traffic accident were recruited. All patients had received a diagnosis of whiplash-associated disorder. Patients with signs of concussion, amnesia, or serious injury (fracture, traumatic internal pathology) were not eligible, and the standard criteria of illiteracy, pregnancy, drug or alcohol abuse, and serious psychopathology were used as exclusion criteria. Using these criteria, two potential participants were excluded, and five men and three women, mean age 45 years (SD = 10.30 years), mean duration of pain 44.4 months (range 27.6–67.2 months) were included in the case series. All of the participants had TSK scores greater than 39. Participants used the standard daily diary to record fear of movement/(re)injury, fear of pain, catastrophizing, and pain intensity. They also nominated two activities that represented their main functional goals, for example, working as a nurse, and recorded the difficulty in achieving the activity in the daily diary. They also carried an accelerometer to assess movement, as in the earlier studies. In addition to the daily diary, participants completed the TSK, PHODA, and the Neck Disability Inventory (NDI [7,19,20]) as standardized measures. The two treatment components were 12 one-hour sessions of GE in a 6-week period and 20 one-hour sessions of GA in a 10-week period. The two treatments were provided by different outpatient therapy teams consisting of a behavior therapist and either an occupational therapist or a physical therapist skilled in the cognitive-behavioral rehabilitation of patients with chronic pain.

After a 2-week, no-treatment baseline, participants received either GE followed by GA or the reverse sequence of treatments. Aggregated responses from the daily diary measures for both treatment sequences are shown in Fig. 9. Visual inspection suggests a clear reduction in all measures,

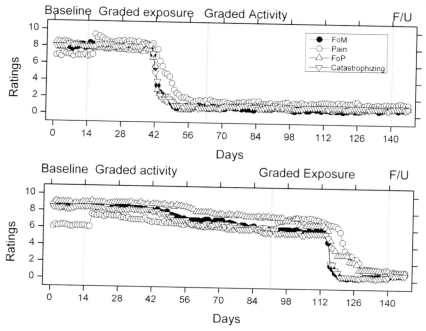

Fig. 9. Aggregated daily diary data for patients in case series 8 in both treatment sequences: baseline–graded exposure (GEXP)–graded activity–follow-up *and* baseline–graded activity–graded exposure–follow-up. Responses on the items measuring fear of movement, pain experience, fear of pain, and pain catastrophizing are shown individually. Redrawn from [3, Fig. 1].

including pain intensity, during GE treatment. These changes occurred 3 to 4 weeks after the start of treatment, and randomization tests confirmed that statistically significant reductions occurred by 5 weeks for all patients, irrespective of the order in which GE was presented (see Table 3 in the original publication). As in the earlier studies, there was little evidence of change during GA when it was presented as the first treatment. Individual responses for nominated functional goals are shown in Fig. 10. Changes in these closely mirrored changes in fear of movement, fear of pain, catastrophizing, and pain intensity and they also showed evidence of a significant statistical change by the end of treatment. The standard measures also reflected these changes, with reductions in TSK means from greater than 40 to 23 or 24 after GE. The PHODA scores were reduced, from greater than 80 to less than 10 for each treatment sequence, and scores on the NDI were reduced from ~30 to less than 10 after GE. The accelerometry

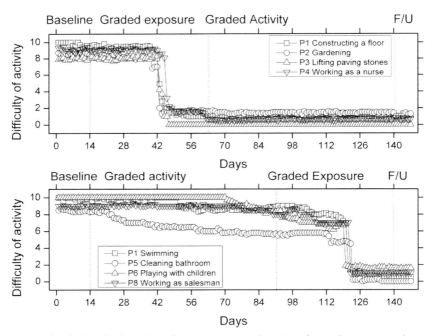

Fig. 10. Individual daily dairy data for one nominated activity for each patient in the two treatment sequences in case study 8: baseline–graded exposure (GEXP)–graded activity–follow-up *and* baseline–graded activity–graded exposure–follow-up. The visual analogue scale records the daily difficult in engaging in the activity (10 = "impossible," 0 = "no problem at all"). Redrawn from [3, Fig. 2].

data also reflected this pattern of change, with marked increases occurring with the introduction of GE. As in the earlier studies, there was less effect on these measures for GA when it was presented first (see Table 2 in the original publication).

Summary of the Case Series

With one exception, in which repeated measures necessary for a single-case experiment could not be obtained (case series 4), seven case series show evidence that the subjective reports of the central components of fear of movement, fear of pain, and catastrophizing were markedly reduced when GE was introduced. When a bona fide comparator treatment, GA, was delivered there was little evidence that comparable reductions in reported fear were achieved. The studies also demonstrated that the treatment could be generalized to a different health care system, different therapists, and to two conditions other than chronic low back pain. Where data on behavioral performance and movement were obtained, this indicated that the reduction of fear was accompanied by specific behavioral changes. Other measures of self-report that assessed the broader concept of disability, for example, the RDQ also indicated that significant behavioral change had occurred.

The case series were also able to explore the possible contribution of the educational component of GE and the role of the patients' perceptions of treatment credibility and the expectation of treatment gain. The evidence for both of these factors was undeniably mixed. In studies in which patients had musculoskeletal pain, there was evidence that the highly structured and personalized education session, during which the patient was presented with the specific case formulation (conceptualization) integral to GE, resulted in a modest reduction of the patient's fear report. However, in the case series of patients with CRPS-I, the education intervention had no effect whatsoever. A major difference between these two conditions was that whereas the patients with musculoskeletal pain rated the treatment as credible and had a positive therapeutic expectation, patients with CRPS-I were skeptical and pessimistic about the efficacy of the treatment. Therefore, it is possible that the education effect might be attributed to the concurrent effect of perceived credibility and expectation of therapeutic gain. However, one case series showed that even though perceived credibility and expectations were the same for GE and GA, change only occurred in the GE phase, suggesting that credibility alone is not a sufficient explanation.

References

[1]   Barlow DH, Nock M, Hersen M. Single case experimental designs: strategies for studying behavior change. New York: Pearson; 2009.
[2]   Boersma K, Linton S, Overmeer T, Jansson M, Vlaeyen J, de Jong J. Lowering fear-avoidance and enhancing function through exposure in vivo. A multiple baseline study across six patients with back pain. Pain 2004;108:8–16.
[3]   de Jong JR, Vangronsveld K, Peters ML, Goossens ME, Onghena P, Bulte I, Vlaeyen JW. Reduction of pain-related fear and disability in post-traumatic neck pain: a replicated single-case experimental study of exposure in vivo. J Pain 2008;9:1123–34.
[4]   de Jong JR, Vlaeyen JWS, Onghena P, Cuypers C, den Hollander M, Ruijgrok J. Reduction of pain-related fear in complex regional pain syndrome type I: the application of graded exposure in vivo. Pain 2005;116:264–75.
[5]   de Jong JR, Vlaeyen JWS, Onghena P, Goossens ME, Geilen M, Mulder H. Fear of movement/(re)injury in chronic low back pain: education or exposure in vivo as mediator to fear reduction? Clin J Pain 2005;21:9–17.
[6]   Fordyce WE. Behavioral methods for chronic pain and illness. St Louis: Mosby; 1976.
[7]   Helmerson AB, Lindgren U. Validity and reliability of a modified version of the neck disability index. J Rehabil Med 2002;34:284–7.
[8]   Kazdin AE. Single case research designs: methods for clinical and applied settings. New York: Oxford University Press; 1982.
[9]   Linton SJ, Hallden K. Can we screen for problematic back pain? A screening questionnaire for predicting outcome in acute and subacute back pain. Clin J Pain 1998;14:209–15.
[10] Linton SJ, Overmeer T, Janson M, Vlaeyen JWS, de Jong JR. Graded in-vivo exposure treatment for fear-avoidant pain patients with functional disability: a case study. Cogn Behav Ther 2002;31:49–58.
[11] Morley S. Single case research. In: Parry G, Watts FN, editors. Behavioural and mental health research: a handbook of skills and methods. Hove: Lawrence Erlbaum Associates; 1996. p. 277–314.
[12] Oerlemans HM, Cup EH, DeBoo T, Goris RJ, Oostendorp RA. The Radboud skills questionnaire: construction and reliability in patients with reflex sympathetic dystrophy of one upper extremity. Disabil Rehabil 2000;22:233–45.
[13] Riley JF, Ahern DK, Follick MJ. Chronic pain and functional impairment: assessing beliefs about their relationship. Arch Phys Med Rehabil 1988;69:579–82.
[14] Roelofs J, Peters ML, Muris P, Vlaeyen JWS. Dutch version of the Pain Vigilance and Awareness Questionnaire: validity and reliability in a pain-free population. Behav Res Ther 2002;40:1081–90.
[15] Roorda LD, Molenaar IW, Lankhorst GJ, Bouter LM. Improvement of a questionnaire measuring activity limitations in rising and sitting down in patients with lower-extremity disorders living at home. Arch Phys Med Rehabil 2005;86:2204–10.
[16] Roorda LD, Roebroeck ME, Lankhorst GJ, van Tilburg T, Bouter LM. Measuring functional limitations in rising and sitting down: development of a questionnaire. Arch Phys Med Rehabil 1996;77:663–9.
[17] Roorda LD, Roebroeck ME, van Tilburg T, Lankhorst GJ, Bouter LM. Measuring activity limitations in climbing stairs: development of a hierarchical scale for patients with lower-extremity disorders living at home. Arch Phys Med Rehabil 2004;85:967–71.
[18] Sidman M. The tactics of scientific research. New York: Basic Books; 1960.
[19] Vernon H. The Neck Disability Index: state-of-the-art, 1991–2008. J Manipulative Physiol Ther 2008;31:491–502.

[20] Vernon H, Mior S. The Neck Disability Index: a study of reliability and validity. J Manipulative Physiol Ther 1991;14:409–15.
[21] Vlaeyen JW, de Jong J, Geilen M, Heuts PH, van Breukelen G. Graded exposure in vivo in the treatment of pain-related fear: a replicated single-case experimental design in four patients with chronic low back pain. Behav Res Ther 2001;39:151–66.
[22] Vlaeyen JW, De Jong JR, Onghena P, Kerckhoffs-Hanssen M, Kole-Snijders AM, Vlaeyen JWS, De Jong JR, Onghena P, Kerckhoffs-Hanssen M, Kole-Snijders AMJ. Can pain-related fear be reduced? The application of cognitive-behavioural exposure in vivo. Pain Res Manag 2002;7:144–53.
[23] Vlaeyen JWS, de Jong J, Geilen M, Heuts PHTG, Breukelen Gv. The treatment of fear of movement/(re)injury in chronic low back pain: Further evidence on the effectiveness of exposure in vivo. Clin J Pain 2002;18:251–61.
[24] Von Korff M, Moore JE, Lorig K, Cherkin DC, Saunders K, Gonzalez VM, Laurent D, Rutter C, Comite F. A randomized trial of a lay person-led self-management group intervention for back pain patients in primary care. Spine 1998;23:2608–15.
[25] Waddell G, Newton M, Henderson I, Somerville D, Main CJ. A fear-avoidance beliefs questionnaire (FABQ) and the role of fear-avoidance beliefs in chronic low-back-pain and disability. Pain 1993;52:157–68.

Randomized Controlled Trials

Whatever the merits of single-case series, they are regarded as less valuable than randomized controlled trials (RCTs), which provide the gold standard in evidence-based practice because of their capacity to control for biases that cannot be controlled for in single-case studies. Because RCTs require larger sample sizes, they can also establish that the effects of treatment are robust and not based merely on exceptional circumstances or responses from a few patients.

We are aware of three relatively small RCTs that have used the graded exposure (GE) treatment protocol described in the previous chapters. All of the studies were published within a few months of each other in 2008; two were the result of work carried out in Sweden [8] and The Netherlands [7] by various authors of this book, and the third [15] was conducted in Canada somewhat independent of the group that developed the treatment. The three trials vary somewhat with respect to design, control groups, and measures used to assess outcome. Two trials [8,15] included a wait-list control condition. This comparison tests the *absolute efficacy* of the treatment, that is, whether it is more effective than no treatment. Trials reported by Leeuw and colleagues [7] and Woods and Asmundson [15] also included graded activity (GA) as an active treatment control. This comparison provided evidence of the *relative efficacy* of GE as a treatment. The expectation generated from the

single-case studies is that graded in vivo exposure (GE) is more effica-
cious than GA.

We start our review of the RCTs by examining the trial reported
by Woods and Asmundson [15]. They randomized 83 participants into
two treatment groups, GE ($n = 36$), GA ($n = 25$), and a wait-list control
group (WLC; $n = 22$). Participants were recruited from advertisements
in the community and posters placed in hospitals and physiotherapist
offices. A total of 151 individuals answered the advertisements; 63 were
excluded at screening, and an additional five dropped out before randomization. Eligibility criteria were a Tampa Scale for Kinesiophobia
(TSK) score of 38 or greater, no pending medical investigations for back
pain, not undergoing other physiotherapy or psychotherapy, and age 18
to 65 years. Of the 83 randomized participants, 39 dropped out of the
trial (GE, $n = 21$; GA, $n = 12$; WLC, $n = 6$). The proportion of dropouts
in the GE group was greater than that in the WLC group, but other comparisons between groups were not significant. The authors noted that
most of the attrition occurred before the initial detailed assessment or
first treatment session but after the participants had been informed of
treatment allocation.

There were a number of marked differences between this trial and
the single-case series. First, the primary outcome measure was the Pain
Disability Index (PDI) [12]. This tool is a short, seven-item questionnaire
that is not specific to back pain, and although it purports to have acceptable psychometric qualities, it is not generally used in trials. The other
measures included the Hospital Anxiety and Depression Scale (HADS
[16]), the short form of the McGill Pain Questionnaire (SF-MPQ) [9],
and the Pain Self-Efficacy Questionnaire (PSEQ) [10]. Measures of fear
avoidance included the TSK, Pain Anxiety Symptoms Scale (PASS), Pain
Catastrophizing Scale (PCS), and Fear-Avoidance Beliefs Questionnaire
(FABQ) used in the single-case studies. Perceived treatment credibility
was also measured. The second difference between this trial and the previous single-case studies was that GE was delivered in eight sessions over a
4-week period, for a total of 6 hours. The first of these sessions comprised
assessment with the Photograph Series of Daily Activities (PHODA) and
education. A single clinical psychologist performed all of the sessions.
In previous studies, GE had been administered by a team comprising a

physiotherapist and a psychologist. The GA therapy was administered by a physiotherapist.

Neither the intent-to-treat (all patients entering the trial irrespective of whether they completed treatment) nor the per-protocol (only those who completed treatment) analyses found a significant effect of treatment on the primary outcome variable (the PDI). Significant differences between the treatments were found for the TSK and PCS posttreatment by intent-to-treat analysis. Further analyses showed that compared to the WLC group, participants receiving GE made greater improvements on several measures (TSK, PCS, FABQ, HADS, and SF-MPQ). Woods and Asmundson [15] also used the Clinically Significant Change method to determine the number of participants making a clinically significant change. They noted that whereas it would have been preferable to have conducted this analysis on the PDI data, this presented a problem because the means scores were "too low and the standard deviations too high." As an alternative, the TSK data were analyzed, and this analysis showed that a greater proportion of participants in the GE group made clinically significant changes than in either of the other groups.

The results of this trial are far from clear. The intent-to-treat analysis did reveal a treatment effect on two of the fear measures (TSK and PCS), but there was no effect on the primary outcome measure (PDI), and there was no evidence for substantial differences between the two treatment arms of the trial. Per-protocol and subsidiary analyses did reveal marginal differences between the two active treatment arms on a measure of self-efficacy (PSEQ); however, this finding was not particularly specific with regard to the purported active mechanisms of GE and we should exercise caution given the more substantive problem of the small size and lack of statistical power of the trial. As noted earlier, the choice of PDI as the primary outcome was problematic with respect to its robustness as a primary outcome measure. The mean PDI score at the start of treatment was ~20, and compared to other clinical data, this score appeared rather low and suggested that the participants, while reporting disability, were not extensively disabled. In contrast, evidence for the *absolute* efficacy of GE as a treatment was substantial.

The second small RCT was conducted in Sweden by the same group of researchers that had reported case series 4 and 5 [8]. This trial

compared the GE to a WLC condition and therefore tested only the absolute efficacy of the treatment. Treatment was delivered by four clinical
psychologists, with the support of a physical therapist, for 13 to 15 treatment sessions. The first four of these sessions included assessment, goal
definition, and education. The WLC group was free to follow a treatment
as usual regimen, which was mainly contact with the general practitioner,
analgesics, and physical therapy. At the end of the wait-list period, these
participants were offered GE therapy. Potential participants for the trial
were recruited via referrals from primary care physicians, advertisements
in the community, and contact with national insurance offices. Entry criteria were as follows: age 18 to 60 years, spinal pain with limited movement, sick leave because of the problem, a TSK score greater than 35, no
indicators of serious spinal pathology (e.g., cauda equina), and a profile
on the PHODA indicating fear of specific movements. A total of 223 individuals fulfilled the basic criteria and were sent a baseline questionnaire,
149 returned the questionnaire, 70 of these were excluded because their
TSK score was less than 35, and an additional 33 were excluded because of
constraints on therapist resources, leaving a final group of 46 individuals
who were randomized to the two treatment arms. Of the 21 individuals
assigned to GE, 13 completed end-of-treatment assessments. Of the eight
dropouts, only one explicitly declined treatment, and the others were excluded or declined for reasons that did not appear to be related to the
treatment per se. A similar pattern of dropout occurred in the WLC group.

No primary outcome measure was explicitly declared in this trial,
but the authors did use the Quebec Back Pain Disability Scale (QBPDS) [5]
as the measure of disability as well as an activities of daily living (ADL) scale
that was designed for the study. Measures of pain-related fear included
the TSK, PCS, and PHODA. The authors conducted both a per-protocol
analysis of the data and a series of intent-to-treat analyses in which they
imputed the missing data for best, worst, and intermediate case scenarios.
This methodology made for difficulty in attempting to review the results.
At one extreme (worst-case scenario), the results were the simplest: no
differences between either of the groups for any of the measures. In contrast, the best-case analysis showed effects for the QBPDS, ADL scale,
TSK, and PCS. The per-protocol analysis revealed an effect for only the
ADL measure. As with the Woods and Asmundson [15] study, this study

was limited by the sample size and lack of statistical power of the analysis, and an unambiguous statement regarding the absolute effectiveness of GE could not be made. However, it was possible to compare the pre- to post-treatment and 3-month follow-up scores for all 23 participants (combined GE and WLC) completing the GE protocol on the TSK, PCS, and PHODA (see Table 4 in the original publication) with the data obtained from the single-case studies. The feature of this comparison was that not only were the pre-post effects smaller, the mean pretreatment scores on these measures were notably lower. This finding was not unexpected given that a selection criterion for entry into the trial was a TSK score of 35 or greater compared with a cut-off score of 39 of 40 in the single-case series. The authors also noted that a proportion of participants with high TSK scores had little or no fear-related activity when this was assessed in more detail with the PHODA. This result suggests that for the treatment to be effective, it should be specifically targeted to those with high levels of fear *and* low levels of function.

The third study [7] was a multicenter trial that included the Dutch treatment facility where several of the single-case studies were performed. With one exception, staff members were employed by the treatment centers. The exception was a clinical psychologist appointed to the trial who treated approximately half of the patients across three of the treatment centers. Teams of therapists comprising a combination of clinical psychologists, occupational therapists, and physical therapists were formed at each of four centers. Various permutations comprised 19 miniteams that treated 1 to 12 patients. Each team was trained to deliver both GE and GA treatment. Treatment manuals were created, and team supervision was performed three times a year. The GE treatment consisted of 16 one-hour sessions, and the GA treatment consisted of 26 one-hour sessions.

Patients with chronic low back pain were recruited from physician referrals and from responses to advertisements in the community. Inclusion criteria included pain for more than 3 years, age 18 to 65 years, no serious spinal injury, Roland-Morris Disability Questionnaire (RDQ) score greater than 3, and a TSK score greater than 33. (Note that this criterion was one standard deviation [SD] below the TSK score of <39 used in the initial studies.) Exclusion criteria were pregnancy, illiteracy, substance abuse, ongoing litigation, medical disorder preventing exercise, or serious psychopathology. The a priori power analysis indicated that a sample of 47 in each group would be needed to provide adequate power for the trial. The teams attempted to recruit 55 individuals into each arm to allow for dropout. In practice, this condition was not met. Of the 177 individuals who were referred to the trial, 85 met the inclusion criteria and were willing to be randomized to one of the treatments; 42 were randomized to GE and 43 to GA. There were 12 dropouts in the GE group (5 because of absence of pain-related fear on further assessment) and 14 dropouts in the GA group.

The primary outcomes for the trial were the QBPDS and, as in the single-case series, patient-specific complaints of three individually nominated activities, each measured on a 100-point visual analog scale (VAS). The secondary outcomes included a shortened version of the PHODA (PHODA-SeV) [6], catastrophizing (PCS), daily activity using a movement monitor as reported in the single-case series, and a measure of pain intensity (100=mm VAS). Analysis of the data included both intent-to-treat and per-protocol methods and were carried out with sophisticated multilevel modeling that adjusted for various confounds.

Immediately after treatment was completed and at the 6-month follow-up, differences between the groups on the QBPDS and patient-specific complaints measures were in the expected direction ($P < 0.10$) but did not meet the predetermined criterion of $P < 0.05$. The GE group did have significantly lower PHODA-SeV and PCS scores at both times, indicating that the intervention did affect the participants' appraisal of pain-related fear. However, there were no significant effects of treatment on recorded activity or pain levels. The analyses were also able to test whether the theoretically specified mediators, that is, reduction in the perceived harmfulness of activity and catastrophizing, were related to outcomes. Initial analysis had shown that the PHODA-SeV and PCS measures changed, and the additional mediation analysis showed that when controlling for treatment arm, both of these measures statistically mediated the outcome, as measured by the QBPDS and patient-related complaints. Although this observation is consistent with the theory, it cannot be read as evidence of causality because there was no temporal lag between the observations [2].

This trial attempted to establish the relative efficacy of GE but found only marginal evidence for the superiority of this treatment. In the absence of a no-treatment control group, we could not be sure that the failure to observe treatment differences was because neither treatment was particularly effective or conversely because both were similarly effective. The authors were able to compare the trial data to that of another large Dutch trial using similar measures that also had a WLC group with similar age and clinical profiles [14]. Comparison with this data demonstrated the superiority of both treatments. Whereas the WLC group showed a gain of 2.65 points (SD = 4.66) on the RDQ, the GA group improved by 4.40 points (SD = 6.13), and the GE group improved by 6.45 points (SD = 5.60). Given that the baseline values were similar across the trials, the observed differences strongly suggest that both GE and GA treatments were effective.

Why was the expected difference between GE and GA not observed in the third trial [7]? The authors' own evaluation of this question [7] highlighted the following possibilities. First, although the number of participants in the trial was considerably larger than those in either the Canadian or Swedish trial, the eventual numbers recruited into the trial were still insufficient to provide adequate power given the a priori power calculation. Second, both treatments share a number of components. Principal among these is exposure to various activities and the provision of explicit reassurance. The major difference is in the selection and sequencing of exposure to the activity. In this study, the same therapeutic teams delivered both treatments. Whereas attempts were made to ensure that the treatments were adhered to and delivered competently [7], it was possible that the educational session in both arms may have been particularly effective in modifying the patients' pain-related beliefs. Third, the GA treatment might have had an advantage because more sessions were administered and the teams were already accustomed to delivering GA, whereas GE was a novel treatment for most members of the team. Fourth, approximately one-third of the participants withdrew from the trial, but as far as could be determined, the reason for terminating treatment was not related to treatment, with the exception of five patients in the GE arm for whom the therapists were unable to determine the presence of fear of movement/(re)injury. This suggests that the TSK cut-off score (33/34) used in the trial might not have been sufficiently stringent to select for patients with a sufficient level of fear. In the series of single-case studies, a

TSK cut-off score of 39 of 40 was used. This score is around the midpoint of the distribution, whereas the 33 of 34 score is one SD below the mean.

Summary

There was a marked contrast between the obvious successes document-ed in the single-case series and the substantially weaker and ambiguous outcomes of the three small RCTs. Why should this be so? One major problem with all of the RCTs was that they were significantly underpow-ered, and even the largest of them [7] had a 20% shortfall of the intended recruitment number. This is critical given that the standard/global out-come measures used are less precise and targeted than the individualized measures used in the single-case studies. Moreover, the major emphasis of the single-case studies was on the measurement of pain-related fear, assessed with daily diary methods, whereas the RCTs focused on stan-dardized measures of disability as the primary outcome assessed on two or three occasions. In addition to the difference in the specificity of the measures, there are two other characteristics that deserve comment. First, we need a better understanding of the relationship between self-reported pain-related fear, measured in the daily diary, and the behavior captured in the various disability measures (RDQ, QBPDS). It is known that changes in subjective fear do not necessarily produce synchronous changes in be-havior and that concordance between affect and behavior may take time to emerge [4,13]. In addition, the specific changes targeted in therapy (e.g., lifting a box, cycling on an uneven surface) might not generalize to the activities specified in the standardized disability measures. Although to be fair, whereas this is a conceptual problem, large changes in the RDQ were observed in the single-case studies. Whether this was attributable to the effect of treatment or to another factor, for example, demand character-istics of the study, remains debatable. Significant changes in measures of pain-related fear on the standardized measures (TSK, PCS, PHODA) were observed in the RCTs, suggesting that the implementation of treatment was associated with the expected reduction of fear.

One notable difference between the single-case series and the RCTs was the frequency of measurement. None of the RCTs required that patients complete a daily diary measure, and we conjecture that the daily monitoring of one's behavior in the context of treatment might be a behavior change mechanism in its own right.

The context in which the two sets of studies were conducted was very different. The majority of the single-case studies were conducted in a specialized Dutch rehabilitation service where participants were resident and where the therapists were the originators and developers of GE and they only delivered GE. In contrast, each of the RCTs was delivered in an outpatient setting where the majority of the therapists were relative novices with regard to GE. Many of the therapists had considerable expertise in other methods, for example GA, for treating chronic pain, and in the trial by Leeuw and colleagues [7], they were required to deliver both treatments. Although Leeuw and colleagues [7] attempted to assess treatment integrity, they could not obtain complete coverage of all therapy teams, and their finding that therapists were adherent to the protocol might have introduced a degree of sampling bias. More importantly, we note that their protocol for assessing adherence could not assess competence in delivering the therapy [7]. This remains a substantive problem that is not specific to this particular therapy [1,3,11]. The possibility that there are significant therapist effects cannot be discounted, and the skill of delivering this treatment should not be underestimated.

Finally, we note that there were substantive differences in selection and attrition between the single-case studies and RCTs. It is notable that all of the trials experienced significant attrition, but it is not clear whether this was specifically associated with the fear-avoidance treatment arm of the trials. There is some evidence for this in Woods and Asmundson's trial [15], but we should note that the numbers were small, and the trial was not powered to detect differential attrition rates. Nevertheless, the presence of attrition should alert us to the need to assess potential participants very carefully with respect to both their general motivation and readiness to engage in therapy and also with respect to their specific suitability for the therapy. This latter issue is particularly salient when we examine the relationship between the cut-off points for the initial screening measure (TSK) and the secondary, more detailed analysis of specific fear-related movements using the PHODA. In the RCTs, several patients were found not to show pain-related fear when the more detailed PHODA assessment was conducted. This finding could be related to the cut-off point on the

TSK used in these trials. Whereas the single-case series used a cutoff score of 39 of 40, two trials used cutoff points that were substantially less than this (35/36 in Linton and colleagues' 2008 study [8], and 33/34 in Leeuw and colleagues' 2008 study [7]). These cutoff points are approximately one SD below the mean of the scale, and when the error of measurement is taken into consideration, it is possible that these trials initially selected patients who were up to two SDs below the mean and would thus be regarded as having very mild fear. As a consequence, the trials might not have been as successful because they failed to select sufficiently fearful patients.

These many subtle differences between the single-case series and the RCTs illustrate some of the complexities of designing and implementing RCTs to test the efficacy of fear-avoidance treatment. The initial trials offer some evidence for the efficacy of the treatment, but there is clearly a need for a large, probably multicenter trial to fully test the treatment model. Meanwhile, the single-case methods reported in this chapter can be implemented in routine practice by competent clinicians at little cost.

References

[1]   Borrelli B, Sepinwall D, Ernst D, Bellg AJ, Czajkowski S, Breger R, DeFrancesco C, Levesque C, Sharp DL, Ogedegbe G, Resnick B, Orwig D. A new tool to assess treatment fidelity and evaluation of treatment fidelity across 10 years of health behavior research. J Consult Clin Psychol 2005;73:852–60.
[2]   Campbell DT, Kenny D. A primer on regression artefacts. New York: Guilford; 1999.
[3]   Gearing RE, El-Bassel N, Ghesquiere A, Baldwin S, Gillies J, Ngeow E. Major ingredients of fidelity: a review and scientific guide to improving quality of intervention research implementation. Clin Psychol Rev 2011;31:79–88.
[4]   Hodgson R, Rachman S. II. Desynchrony in measures of fear. Behav Res Ther 1974;12:319–26.
[5]   Kopec JA, Esdaile JM, Abrahamowicz M, Abenhaim L, Wood-Dauphinee S, Lamping DL, Williams JI. The Quebec Back Pain Disability Scale. Measurement properties. Spine 1995;20:341–52.
[6]   Leeuw M, Goossens ME, van Breukelen GJ, Boersma K, Vlaeyen JW. Measuring perceived harmfulness of physical activities in patients with chronic low back pain: the Photograph Series of Daily Activities—short electronic version. J Pain 2007;8:840–9.
[7]   Leeuw M, Goossens ME, van Breukelen GJ, de Jong JR, Heuts PH, Smeets RJ, Koke AJ, Vlaeyen JW. Exposure in vivo versus operant graded activity in chronic low back pain patients: results of a randomized controlled trial. Pain 2008;138:192–207.
[8]   Linton SJ, Boersma K, Jansson M, Overmeer T, Lindblom K, Vlaeyen JW. A randomized controlled trial of exposure in vivo for patients with spinal pain reporting fear of work-related activities. Eur J Pain 2008;12:722–30.
[9]   Melzack R. The short form McGill Pain Questionnaire. Pain 1987;30:191–7.
[10] Nicholas MK. The pain self-efficacy questionnaire: Taking pain into account. Eur J Pain 2007;11:153–63.
[11] Perepletchikova F, Treat TA, Kazdin AE. Treatment integrity in psychotherapy research: analysis of the studies and examination of the associated factors. J Consult Clin Psychol 2007;75:829–41.
[12] Pollard CA. Preliminary validity study of the Pain Disability Index. Percept Mot Skills 1984;59:974.

[13] Rachman S, Hodgson R. I. Synchrony and desynchrony in fear and avoidance. Behav Res Ther 1974;12:311–8.

[14] Smeets RJ, Vlaeyen JW, Hidding A, Kester AD, van der Heijden GJ, van Geel AC, Knottnerus JA. Active rehabilitation for chronic low back pain: cognitive-behavioral, physical, or both? First direct post-treatment results from a randomized controlled trial [ISRCTN22714229]. BMC Musculoskelet Disord 2006;7:5.

[15] Woods MP, Asmundson GJ. Evaluating the efficacy of graded in vivo exposure for the treatment of fear in patients with chronic back pain: a randomized controlled clinical trial. Pain 2008;136:271–80.

[16] Zigmond AS, Snaith RP. The Hospital Anxiety and Depression Scale. Acta Psychiatr Scand 1983;67:361–70.

Future Directions

In vivo exposure offers an exciting treatment option with considerable potential for relieving suffering for people with chronic pain. Whereas the current outcomes for pain-related fear suggest a promising future, the exposure techniques are nevertheless still under development. The evidence thus far indicates that while exposure is often helpful, it is not successful with every patient nor do most patients experience a full recovery. To meet the full promise of exposure, better procedures that work more uniformly than at present are needed, and to achieve this some unresolved issues need to be addressed. Some of the problems raised in the clinic have clear theoretical underpinnings, while others involve the need to develop further clinical procedures for application. In this chapter, we explore some of the thought-provoking areas in research, assessment, and management of pain-related fear that could be instrumental for scientific advancements and clinical application.

The progress made with exposure treatment has shifted the focus away from a general coping model to a more specific model directed at particular components of experience. Perhaps one of the most important contributions of the fear-avoidance model has been that it emphasizes that specific mechanisms underpinning the relationship between behavior, cognition, and emotion can be tested, and the knowledge gained can be used to develop a treatment. The central feature of exposure treatment is bringing the patient in contact with the feared stimulus without the presence of so-called safety-seeking behavior. Safety-seeking behaviors are things a patient might do to reduce experiencing the stimulus and may include things such as bracing, guarding, and distraction. These actions are unhelpful because they diminish the effects of exposure in that they are also avoidance strategies. The coping approach has been criticized [30,52] because it might appear to encourage safety-seeking behavior. For example, guarding and asking for assistance are commonly employed coping behaviors, but they have been found to be detrimental for patients with fibromyalgia probably because they increase avoidance [21]. Furthermore, coping does not necessarily promote acceptance of the pain and pain-related emotions, as acceptance and commitment therapy (ACT) would advocate. Yet, it might be difficult to engage patients in exposure without coping strategies and it might also be problematic to detect subtle forms of safety-seeking behaviors. As a result, there are several pertinent issues surrounding how exposure is actually construed and conducted. We start by exploring some recent theoretical developments and examine various issues for clinical application, and then proceed to those dealing directly with exposure therapy.

Theoretical Developments

The Predictability of Pain and Pain-Related Anxiety

Although fear conditioning research and its application to pain-related fear has been valuable for understanding chronic regional musculoskeletal pain (such as back, neck, or limb pain), it might not be appropriate for disorders in which the location of pain is more widely distributed and spatially generalized (such as fibromyalgia or complex regional pain syndrome). In musculoskeletal pain, patients are usually quite aware of the contingency between a conditioned stimulus (CS) (e.g., a particular movement) and the unconditioned stimulus (US) (e.g., pain or a pain increase), whereas for widespread pain, patients usually experience an absence of an objective predictor of danger. Current theory predicts that in these cases, because of a lack of apparent safety cues (CS–), experiencing unpredictable pain induces a more general form of distress, demonstrated by feelings of worry and chronic apprehension. This distinction could be important because unpredictability might have an effect on the experienced pain intensity. For example, Rhudy and Meagher [39] tested this experimentally by creating two conditions that differed in the actual delivery of an experimental pain stimulus. In both conditions, participants were told that they might receive brief, surprising, and painful electric shocks. In the fear condition, participants actually received three shocks, whereas in the anxiety condition, they did not receive any shock. The results revealed that fear established by the presentation of shock resulted in greater withdrawal thresholds to subsequent radiant heat, whereas anxiety elicited by anticipation of shock (without actual exposure) decreased pain thresholds. To avoid confounding of a difference in actual pain, Meulders and colleagues [32] used a within-subject design with joystick movements as the CS. Movements in one plane, for example, horizontally, successfully predicted painful shock, whereas those in the other plane (e.g., vertically) were unpaired with shock so that the pain was unpredictable. Results of this study showed that despite an equal number of shocks, both intensity and unpleasantness of the shocks were rated higher in the unpredictable condition compared to the predictable condition. In addition to the increased pain, given the absence of safety cues, it is also likely that pain anxiety (compared to cued fear of pain) is associated with the avoidance of an increased number of stimuli and also stimuli that were never associated with pain in the past. The role of predictable versus unpredictable pain and the effects of different types of (un)predictability (pain duration, pain offset, pain location, pain quality, etc.) clearly warrant more systematic experimental scrutiny and may open a novel window for understanding generalized pain syndromes.

Weighting Pain and Non-pain Goals

Another concern with the current fear-avoidance model relates to the idea that pain-related fear emerges in a context of multiple goals [4,50,51]. The goal of avoiding pain is only one of a number of goals that could be pursued in an environment with concomitant, often competing goals. Indeed, one of the most debilitating consequences of pain-related avoidance behavior is the withdrawal from previously valued activities. In this respect, patients with chronic pain frequently prioritize the value of their pain avoidance against the costs related to the loss of valued activities [40–42].

For example in one study, goal self-efficacy, goal conflict, and pain severity independently predicted pain-induced fear, which in turn mediated the effects of goal conflict on physical disability and depression in patients with chronic low back pain [20]. The idea that pain-related goal conflicts might increase the threat value of the pain is an intriguing one, largely left untested [21].

The Generality of the Fear-Avoidance Model

Thus far, most of the work on pain-related fear has focused on patients with nonspecific medical diagnoses such as back pain, chronic headache [34,37], fibromyalgia [6,48], whiplash disorder [35,47], and chronic fatigue syndrome [36,46]. Theoretically, there is no reason to believe that fear processes would not be applicable to specific pain problems as well. Indeed, the contribution of pain-related fear has shown to extend to patients with hip and knee osteoarthritis [43], burn pain [44], knee injury [23], and neuropathic pain [8] to name a few. Pain-related fear also predicts the outcome of medical procedures such as spinal surgery [1] and arthroscopic knee surgery [19]. It will be a challenge for future researchers to integrate fear reduction techniques in the medical treatment and care of these patient groups.

Clinical Assessment

Although procedures for assessing patients have been described in Chapter 3, challenges remain in more accurately identifying patients appropriate for exposure as well as methods to assist in developing the individual exposure intervention. At the moment, there are clinical recommendations that are helpful. However, the decision to use a certain score on the Tampa Scale for Kinesiophobia (TSK) or the Pain Catastrophizing Scale (PCS) as a criterion is pragmatic. Empirical testing would help us to know exactly which measures are most efficient and what cut-off points might be most appropriate, and further improvements in the reliability of the instruments would enhance their utility. Consequently, more work is needed to develop an assessment battery that would provide essential information for selecting patients. The future will hopefully bring the development of methods to assess patients so that those likely to benefit from exposure can be selected early on. It is particularly appealing to envision a method whereby treatments might be matched to the patient's needs based on, in whole or in part, aspects of the model [45,51].

A second and related aspect is ascertaining what patients are actually afraid of (avoiding) and gauging how intense the fear reaction is. The emotional reaction in pain-related fear is critical for successful exposure, but to date we often struggle to know what the patient fears, for example the pain, a certain movement, or a catastrophe [33]. Ironically, the persistence of attempts to decrease pain may represent the patient's efforts to avoid a broad range of feared-for futures [C. Wells et al., unpublished manuscript]. To date, there is no assessment technique that actually examines the *behavioral avoidance*. A form of a behavioral approach test (BAT), which is typical in the assessment of psychological phobias, would be helpful. It is ironic that the model that focuses on avoidance behavior still has no standardized direct assessment or measure of the actual avoidance. Behavioral approach tests are commonly used with phobias and usually entail asking the patient to approach the feared object, for example a snake, with ratings of fear being made periodically. Behavioral approach tests for pain-related fear could provide clinicians with samples of the patient's avoidance behavior and allow us to better isolate the exact stimuli that elicit the fear response. These might be supplemented with new measures of the emotional reaction. To date, the questionnaires employed (e.g., the TSK and Fear-Avoidance Beliefs Questionnaire [FABQ]) appear to measure beliefs rather than the actual emotional reaction, that is, the fear and worry. During exposure treatment, a simple measure of experienced fear would also be beneficial to gauge whether the exposure is working. The BAT, as well as information from new measures of emotional reactions, would be helpful as part of the psycho-education portion of treatment mentioned below to help the patient understand the nature of the problem and the reason exposure treatment would be relevant.

Finally, standardized methods are needed that allow for better outcome evaluation in the clinic and also for use in formal investigations. Currently, a variety of methods are employed, for example, daily ratings on a few items taken from standardized questionnaires. Whereas these may be helpful, they are not standardized, and their sensitivity is not known. To evaluate outcome, a small set of psychometrically sound measures are needed that clinicians and scientists alike can utilize. Whether this will be achievable is debatable. Readers will recall the discussion in Chapter 6, which distinguished between global/standard measures and target measures. The data from the single-case series (Chapter 7) indicated that specific, patient-centered measures appear to be sensitive outcome measures, whereas the global/standard measures appear to be less sensitive to individual change in the randomized controlled trials (RCTs) reviewed in Chapter 8. The main problem is therefore developing sensitive measures suitable for individuals that can also be referenced to standard norms. In the field of psychometrics, item-response theory offers a potential answer to this problem [12].

Engaging the Patient

Perhaps the biggest challenge facing the implementation of exposure-based treatment for pain-related fear is engaging patients so that they are willing to accept and participate fully in the treatment. Engagement is essential because exposure involves hard work and the likely experience of both pain and negative affect. If patients do not believe or understand the underpinning idea of the treatment, they might easily become concerned or discouraged and refuse or drop out of treatment. Indeed, there are several indicators that patients might not construe their problem as one of emotion and avoidance, and therefore they might have difficulty in engaging in treatment aimed at altering these [18]. Consider the following. First, in a study in preparation, we offered patients one of three different treatments for their musculoskeletal pain problem, graded activity (GA), graded exposure (GE), or a cognitive-behavioral therapy (CBT) package including standard techniques aimed at increasing function and dealing with emotional aspects such as depression. Participants were provided with a brief description of each method and asked which they preferred. The most preferred method was CBT (36%), followed closely by activity training (30%). Some had no preference (20%), but only 14% said they preferred the exposure treatment. Thus, exposure was the least preferred treatment, a finding replicated by George and Robinson [16]. This finding, in conjunction with the worrisome number of dropouts, ranging from ~30% to 58% [24,26,53], might signal a perceived lack of clinical validity and credibility among patients. It could also indicate a failure on the part of the therapist to devise exposure tasks that genuinely expose patients to their fears but that are not overwhelmingly fearful.

To engage patients, new approaches to psycho-education are required. Alternative models for understanding the treatment are desirable. Currently, the model often used in practice is a form of the fear-avoidance model. This model, of course, underscores the role of psychological factors including fear and catastrophizing. Yet, many patients come to us with a strong belief in the need to treat the physiological basis of their pain. Consequently, the fear-avoidance model could be threatening and invalidating because it does not sufficiently mirror their experience. A new model might more appropriately highlight the physiological source of the pain sensation and how they interact with psychological processes. Further, presenting the model in a psycho-educational format could provide some clear guidelines for clinicians on how to judge whether the patient sufficiently understands the model to engage in the treatment.

Second, great advances have been made in the area of patient engagement that could be translated into use in exposure treatment for pain-related fear. These advancements employ various forms of goal-setting as well as other techniques to enhance engagement. The development of goals provides a unique opportunity for increasing engagement. One technique of interest is the use of life values as a framework for developing goals [5,38]. This process involves exploring with patients their personal life values such as the importance of work, family, and leisure activities. Goals are then expounded that are in direct line with these personal values. In this way, the goals should be more enticing for the patient, and engagement should be more profound. By focusing on clear, value-oriented, future goals that involve complex activities, the simple steps in a hierarchy would appear to be more appealing and understandable.

Clinical Application of Exposure

The development of exposure treatment techniques for pain-related fear has been a process marked by swift advances and unexpected obstacles. Applying exposure techniques for pain-related fear requires ingenuity because it is not straightforward to conceive how the CS, for example a movement, can be presented without the US, for example injury. Fortunately, considerable advances have been made, and the techniques described in this book provide a basis for achieving in vivo exposure with such patients. However, there are still a range of issues regarding how exposure might best be developed and applied.

Some attempts have been made to streamline the exposure technique for clinical application. For example, George and colleagues [17] tested a system for GE delivered as a complement to the usual physical therapy delivered by a trained physical therapist. To tease out the additional effects of exposure, a comparison was made with GA. It must be noted, however, that the description of the exposure treatment suggests that this method was significantly different from the procedure described in this book. For example, assessment was performed with a questionnaire containing 10 activities, where the two most feared were selected for exposure. Results showed that the usual physical therapy treatment was not augmented by GA or GE, a finding that surprised the authors. This is intriguing because in vivo exposure needs to be tested against other active treatments, and attempts to test whether perceived harmfulness of the activities diminished were lacking. It also suggests that true exposure may not have been achieved, underscoring that whereas new methods are needed to facilitate better results and application, care is required to preserve the fidelity of the method.

New Methods of Delivery

Competent delivery of in vivo exposure is challenging for both the patient and the therapist. A basic dilemma in exposure therapy, as mentioned above, is discovering what the feared CS is and then being able to present it without the presence of the injury/pain (US) [33]. Many patients with persistent pain problems have more or less continuous pain. Thus, some of the stimuli triggering the fear response may be internal stimuli in the form of the pain itself or proprioceptive stimuli arising from movement [9]. How might these stimuli be utilized in exposure? In addition, in vivo exposure is only one type of exposure; modeling and verbal instruction might also be effective methods. There is a clear need to develop new methods and ideas concerning the delivery of exposure treatment. For example, interoceptive exposure might be one method of dealing with the internal stimuli, for example the pain itself or the proprioceptive stimuli arising from movement that triggers the fear. One study [13] has examined the potential of interceptive exposure by asking patients with chronic pain to practice focusing on the persistent pain using a regular practice schedule. The study used a case-series design, and the results are encouraging, but the method clearly requires further practical and theoretical development [9].

New methods could also take advantage of advances being made in CBT. ACT has been used with patients with various forms of persistent pain [28,49]. The technique is interesting for exposure for several reasons. First, an emphasis in ACT is on experiencing bodily sensations, thoughts, and feelings without judging them, such as in mindfulness. This has direct implications for dealing with so-called safety-seeking behaviors during exposure. These behaviors, as described above, are subtle ways of avoiding the fear and bodily sensations during exposure, and there is some evidence that these behaviors hinder the fear extinction process. A focus on experiencing the sensations and feelings, rather than avoiding them, might have value by enhancing the exposure treatment [10]. Second, ACT also focuses on the concept of behavioral flexibility [29]. The misdirected problem-solving model of chronic pain highlights the clinical observation that many patients with pain become rigid and see only a few options for dealing with (solving) their pain problem [11; C. Wells et al., unpublished manuscript]. This situation might affect exposure because the behaviors we ask patients to perform may be new ones. Methods that enhance flexibility should facilitate engagement and performance. Third, ACT uses various aspects of exposure in treatment incorporating modeling and information. Whereas there are several studies demonstrating that an ACT approach to pain is associated with improvements [31], a recent systematic review suggests that ACT is effective, but not more so than other behavioral treatments [49] and that it may provide for important alternative treatment options. Therefore, there is a need to study how this approach might best be utilized to achieve exposure.

Dialectical behavior therapy (DBT) is yet another development within CBT that brings potentially useful ideas to the arena. First, DBT underscores the role of emotions and difficulties in regulating emotions as strong forces in many problems [14,25]. This aspect is particularly relevant because exposure in fact is designed to help patients "regulate" their fear and worry. Dialectical behavior therapy (DBT) draws on a number of other emotion regulation strategies that could be useful for the development of exposure techniques. Unlike ACT or CBT, the use of emotion regulation strategies, which sooth negative affect, are employed in DBT as a way of assisting the patient in achieving exposure. Second, DBT extensively uses validation as a method of obtaining good communication and engagement, which are necessary components for good psycho-education and goal-setting [3,15]. Validation relates to actively making statements that acknowledge the truth of the feelings, thoughts, and experiences of the patient. Validation shows that the clinician is listening, interested, and accepts the patient's experiences as real. It has been shown to have a soothing effect on emotions and to decrease worry about pain in experimental studies [27]. It has also been implicated as an important factor for engagement in therapy [27]. To date, however, we do not know how validation or other emotion regulation techniques might influence exposure. Such techniques would appear to have considerable potential for communication, preparation, engagement, and actual exposure. Third, DBT works actively with "opposites" such that one can accept something but also strive for change. This tool might be helpful in psycho-education; the need to accept certain aspects of the pain but at the same time striving to alter other aspects such as the emotional and functional consequences. The idea of opposites could also provide impetus for selecting exposure activities, especially when generalizing to natural settings. In a nutshell, like flexibility (above), the idea of opposites can assist the patient in seeing that there are other behaviors that might be appropriate such as approaching (exposure) rather than avoiding. Whereas DBT has demonstrated success with some difficult emotional and psychological problems, such as borderline personality disorder [22], only one case study has explored its use as a way of enhancing exposure [25]. Thus, while DBT has relevance, much research is needed to explore its potential contribution to this area.

From the Clinic to Routine Everyday Life

Generalizing improvements made in the clinic to the home or work environment, as well as from one feared movement to another, is of fundamental importance. In short, we might wonder how well patients can take what they have learned during treatment and apply it to their everyday life. This involves generalizing from the clinic to other environments such as home or work. In addition, because patients may experience various degrees of pain-related fear for a host of movements, there is a question as to whether they can generalize what they have learned for one movement and apply it on their own to another. These central issues have ramifications for long-term maintenance of treatment gains because difficulties with generalization will undermine long-term effects.

As we saw in Chapter 4, clinicians are encouraged to enhance generalization by using various techniques. First, providing relevant homework between sessions should help generalize the effects from the clinic to other environments. This usually involves practicing the movement in an everyday situation. For example, a patient with fear related to reaching and stretching might be given an assignment to reach and stretch to take cups from the shelf when setting the table. These kinds of homework are believed to be instrumental in promoting generalization. Second, clinicians are also encouraged to progress from one movement to another, which ought to promote generalization of the technique from one type of movement to another. Recently, it has been found that using multiple stimuli during the exposure treatment can enhance generalization [7]. There is a need, however, to study how well transfer from the clinic to everyday life occurs and to explore new techniques to enhance generalization and maintenance of the effects. These might focus on in-clinic training, for example how the stimuli are presented, but could also entail homework assignments and developing goals underscoring daily life.

Clinical Translation

Perhaps the greatest challenge for the future is applying our knowledge about in vivo exposure to standard clinical practice. Indeed, the question immediately arises as to how this might best be accomplished, that is, how do we identify patients, who should conduct the treatment, and when and where should it be delivered. There appear to be at least two parts to this issue. The first centers on identifying and treating those patients who clearly would be expected to benefit from in vivo exposure treatment. As mentioned above, clinical assessment methods are needed, but while necessary, they are in themselves not sufficient to obtain a system for identifying these patients. We envision that secondary, specialist pain rehabilitation services would routinely assess patients who may likely benefit. The flip side would be a program to provide in vivo exposure in a setting that truly supports this approach, for example with consistent messages from every professional. The past 10 years of research have certainly seen a shift in the approach to pain rehabilitation from a more general coping approach to a more specific fear-avoidance approach, and the future should bring an application of this to the clinic.

The second issue concerns early intervention, which might prevent the development of disability owing to pain-related fear. Addressing pain-related fear early on might well be helpful in preventing its further exacerbation leading to disability. Further work is needed to develop a system for identifying these patients and then providing appropriate early treatment. Considerable advances have been made in screening for patients who will likely develop problems [2], and these patients may deserve further assessment. However, it is doubtful whether this routinely happens in today's clinical reality. Once a patient is identified early on, there is a need for an intervention that targets the problem. Whereas GA and other activation programs have been put forward to fill this need, research is required to evaluate and further develop interventions. For example, GA may not be specific enough, while in vivo exposure might be unnecessary. Our sense is that if we can assess at the primary care level so that we can identify patients who experience pain-related fear and avoidance, exposure techniques should be effective. Achieving excellent assessment and proper treatment routinely in first-line settings, for example in primary care, involves imminent challenges.

The Way Forward

A solid base for in vivo exposure has been laid, providing a rich source for theoretical and clinical reflection. Much has been achieved. We now have knowledge and methods about the mechanisms involved, which has paved the way for assessment and treatment techniques. Yet much remains to be done. First, there is the vision of making the assessment and treatment techniques widely available so that patients with pain-related fear might be helped at an appropriate juncture. This underscores the dire need for translating new knowledge into clinical routines so that patients everywhere might benefit. Concurrent evidence for the effectiveness of exposure needs to be acquired so that we can select the most relevant and effective treatment methods. The techniques for assessment and treatment described in this book are basic, and one way forward is to develop and test them further to enhance their efficiency and efficacy.

Second, treatment might better engage the patient and target specific needs. The way forward is via better assessment methods, which pinpoint more exactly pertinent mechanisms, as well as better methods of explaining the relevance of the treatment to patients. We envision methods for providing psycho-education and communicating with patients that use the patients' own resources and ignite their interest and enthusiasm. Because exposure is a very challenging method, this would provide a clear step forward.

Third, research on basic mechanisms and variations of exposure could open new doors to success. To fully utilize the power of exposure, basic research is needed to explore the learning base upon which exposure rests. We foresee laboratory and clinical studies that elucidate the fundamental processes involved. Moreover, we foresee investigations of novel approaches to the application of exposure that might enhance its benefits and increase its generalization to larger groups of patients.

Much hard work has been done. Shifting focus toward pain-related fear has provided a clear step forward in our understanding and treatment of pain problems. With these advances, clinical application is now not only possible, but recommended. Yet, we cannot rest. Whereas the base of knowledge that we now have provides a worthy platform for treatment, tomorrow's needs demand the launching of theoretical, experimental, treatment outcome, and clinical application studies. We look forward to reaping the benefits.

References

[1] Archer K, Wegener S, Seebach C, Skolasky R, Thornton C, Khanna J, Riley LH 3rd. Fear-avoidance beliefs on pain intensity and patient-reported disability after spine surgery. Arch Phys Med Rehabil 2009;90:e3.
[2] Boersma K, Linton SJ. Screening to identify patients at risk: profiles of psychological risk factors for early intervention. Clin J Pain 2005;21:38–43; discussion 69–72.
[3] Cano A, Williams ACC. Social interaction in pain: reinforcing pain behaviors or building intimacy? Pain 2010;149:9–11.

[4]   Crombez G, Eccleston C, Van Damme S, Vlaeyen JW, Karoly P. The fear avoidance model of chronic pain: the next generation. Clin J Pain 2012; 2012;28:275–83.

[5]   Dahl JAC, Plumb J, Stewart I, Lundgren T. The art and science of valuing in psychotherapy: helping clients discover, explore, and commit to valued action using acceptance and commitment therapy. New Harbinger; 2009.

[6]   de Gier M, Peters ML, Vlaeyen JW. Fear of pain, physical performance, and attentional processes in patients with fibromyalgia. Pain 2003;104:121–30.

[7]   de Jong J, den Hollander M, Bulté I, Ruijgrok J, Vlaeyen J. Generalization of graded exposure in vivo in complex regional pain syndrome type I. Pain; in revision.

[8]   de Jong J, Vlaeyen JWS, de Gelder JM, Patijn J. Pain-related fear, perceived harmfulness of activities, and functional limitations in complex regional pain syndrome type I. J Pain 2011;12:1209–18.

[9]   De Peuter S, Van Diest I, Vansteenwegen D, Van den Bergh O, Vlaeyen JW. Understanding fear of pain in chronic pain: interoceptive fear conditioning as a novel approach. Eur J Pain 2011;15:889–94.

[10] den Hollander M, de Jong JR, Volders S, Goossens ME, Smeets RJ, Vlaeyen JWS. Fear reduction in patients with chronic pain: a learning theory perspective. Expert Rev Neurother 2010;10:1733–45.

[11] Eccleston C, Crombez G. Worry and chronic pain: a misdirected problem solving model. Pain 2007;132:233–6.

[12] Embretson SE, Reise S. Item response theory for psychologists. Mahwah, NJ: Erlbaum; 2000.

[13] Flink I, Nicholas M, Boersma K, Linton S. Reducing the threat value of chronic pain: a preliminary replicated single-case study of interoceptive exposure versus distraction in six individuals with chronic back pain. Behav Res Ther 2009;47:721–8.

[14] Fruzzetti AE, Crook W, Erikson K, Lee J, Worrall JM. Emotion regulation. In: O'Donohue WT, Fisher JE, editors. General principles and empirically supported techniques of cognitive behavior therapy. Hoboken, NJ: Wiley; 2009. p. 272–84.

[15] Fruzzetti AE, Worrall JM. Accurate expression and validation: a transactional model for understanding individual and relationship distress. In: Sullivan K, Davila J, editors. Support processes in intimate relationships. Oxford: Oxford University Press, 2010.

[16] George SZ, Robinson ME. Preference, expectation, and satisfaction in a clinical trial of behavioral interventions for acute and sub-acute low back pain. J Pain 2010;11:1074–82.

[17] George SZ, Zeppieri Jr G, Cere AL, Cere MR, Borut MS, Hodges MJ, Reed DM, Valencia C, Robinson ME. A randomized trial of behavioral physical therapy interventions for acute and sub-acute low back pain. Pain 2008;140:145–57.

[18] Hadjistavropoulos HD, Kowalyk KM. Patient-therapist relationships among patients with pain-related fear. In: Asmundson GJ, Vlaeyen JWS, Crombez G, editors. Understanding and treating fear of pain. Oxford: Oxford University Press; 2004. p. 237–64.

[19] Johansson A, Cornefjord M, Bergkvist L, Öhrvik J, Linton S. Psychosocial stress factors among patients with lumbar disc herniation, scheduled for disc surgery in comparison with patients scheduled for arthroscopic knee surgery. Eur Spine J 2007;16:961–70.

[20] Karoly P, Okun MA, Ruehlman LS, Pugliese JA. The impact of goal cognition and pain severity on disability and depression in adults with chronic pain: an examination of direct effects and mediated effects via pain-induced fear. Cognit Ther Res 2008;32:418–33.

[21] Karsdorp PA, Vlaeyen JW. Goals matter: both achievement and pain-avoidance goals are associated with pain severity and disability in patients with low back and upper extremity pain. Pain 2011;152:1382–90.

[22] Kliem S, Kröger C, Kosfelder J. Dialectical behavior therapy for borderline personality disorder: a meta-analysis using mixed-effects modeling. J Consult Clin Psychol 2010;78:936.

[23] Kvist J, Ek A, Sporrstedt K, Good L. Fear of re-injury: a hindrance for returning to sports after anterior cruciate ligament reconstruction. Knee Surg Sports Traumatol Arthrosc 2005;13:393–7.

[24] Leeuw M, Goossens M, Van Breukelen G, De Jong J, Heuts PH, Smeets R. Exposure in vivo versus operant graded activity in chronic low back pain patients: results of a randomized controlled trial. Pain 2008;138:192–207.

[25] Linton SJ. Applying dialectical behavior therapy to chronic pain: a case study. Scand J Pain 2010;1:50–4.

[26] Linton SJ, Boersma K, Jansson M, Overmeer T, Lindblom K, Vlaeyen JWS. A randomized controlled trial of exposure in vivo for patients with spinal pain reporting fear of work-related activities. Eur J Pain 2008;12:722–30.

[27] Linton SJ, Boersma K, Vangronsveld K, Fruzzetti A. Painfully reassuring? The effects of validation on emotions and adherence in a pain test. Eur J Pain 2012;16:592–9.

[28] McCracken LM. Contextual cognitive-behavioral therapy for chronic pain. Seattle: IASP Press; 2005.

[29] McCracken LM. Mindfulness and acceptance in behavioral medicine: current theory and practice. Oakland, CA: Context Press; 2011.

[30] McCracken LM, Eccleston C. Coping or acceptance: what to do about chronic pain? Pain 2003;105:197–204.

[31] McCracken LM, Gauntlett-Gilbert J. Role of psychological flexibility in parents of adolescents with chronic pain: development of a measure and preliminary correlation analyses. Pain 2011;152:780–5.

[32] Meulders A, Vansteenwegen D, Vlaeyen JW. The acquisition of fear of movement-related pain and associative learning: a novel pain-relevant human fear conditioning paradigm. Pain 2011;152:2460–9.

[33] Morley S, Eccleston C. The object of fear in pain. In: Asmundson GJ, Vlaeyen JWS, Crombez G, editors. Understanding and treating fear of pain. Oxford: Oxford University Press; 2004. p. 163–88.

[34] Nash JM, Williams DM, Nicholson R, Trask PC. The contribution of pain-related anxiety to disability from headache. J Behav Med 2006;29:61–7.

[35] Nederhand MJ, Ijzerman MJ, Hermens HJ, Turk DC, Zilvold G. Predictive value of fear avoidance in developing chronic neck pain disability: consequences for clinical decision making. Arch Phys Med Rehabil 2004;85:496–501.

[36] Nijs J, De Meirleir K, Duquet W. Kinesiophobia in chronic fatigue syndrome: assessment and associations with disability. Arch Phys Med Rehabil 2004;85:1586–92.

[37] Norton PJ, Asmundson GJ. Anxiety sensitivity, fear, and avoidance behavior in headache pain. Pain 2004;111:218–23.

[38] Plumb JC, Stewart I, Dahl JA, Lundgren T. In search of meaning: values in modern clinical behavior analysis. Behav Anal 2009;32:85.

[39] Rhudy JL, Meagher MW. Fear and anxiety: divergent effects on human pain thresholds. Pain 2000;84:65–75.

[40] Roy M. Weighting pain avoidance and reward seeking: a neuroeconomical approach to pain. J Neurosci 2010;30:4185–6.

[41] Schrooten MG, Vlaeyen JW. Becoming active again? Further thoughts on goal pursuit in chronic pain. Pain 2010;149:422–3.

[42] Schrooten MGS, Vlaeyen JWS, Morley S. Psychological interventions for chronic pain: reviewed within the context of goal pursuit. Pain Manag 2012;2:1–10.

[43] Scopaz K, Piva SR, Wisniewski S, GK. F. Relationships of fear, anxiety, and depression with physical function in patients with knee osteoarthritis. Arch Phys Med Rehabil 2009;90:1866–73.

[44] Sgroi MI, Willebrand M, Ekselius L, Gerdin B, Andersson G. Fear-avoidance in recovered burn patients: association with psychological and somatic symptoms. J Health Psychol 2005;10:491–502.

[45] Shaw WS, Linton SJ, Pransky G. Reducing sickness absence from work due to low back pain: how well do intervention strategies match modifiable risk factors? J Occup Rehabil 2006;16:591–605.

[46] Silver A, Haeney M, Vijayadurai P, Wilks D, Pattrick M, Main CJ. The role of fear of physical movement and activity in chronic fatigue syndrome. J Psychosom Res 2002;52:485–93.

[47] Sterling M, Kenardy J, Jull G, Vicenzino B. The development of psychological changes following whiplash injury. Pain 2003;106:481–9.

[48] Turk DC, Robinson JP, Burwinkle T. Prevalence of fear of pain and activity in patients with fibromyalgia syndrome. J Pain 2004;5:483–90.

[49] Veehof MM, Oskam MJ, Schreurs KM, Bohlmeijer ET. Acceptance-based interventions for the treatment of chronic pain: a systematic review and meta-analysis. Pain 2011;152:533–42.

[50] Vlaeyen JWS, Crombez G, Linton SJ. The fear-avoidance model of pain: we are not there yet. Comment on Wideman et al. "A prospective sequential analysis of the fear-avoidance model of pain" [Pain, 2009] and Nicholas "First things first: reduction in catastrophizing before fear of movement" [Pain, 2009]. Pain 2009;146:222.

[51] Vlaeyen JWS, Morley S. Introduction to Special Issue. Clin J Pain 2005;21:1–8.

[52] Vowles KE, Thompson M. Acceptance and commitment therapy for chronic pain. In: McCracken L, editor. Mindfulness and acceptance in behavioral medicine. Oakland, CA: Context Press; 2011. p. 31–60.

[53] Woods MP, Asmundson GJ. Evaluating the efficacy of graded in vivo exposure for the treatment of fear in patients with chronic back pain: a randomized controlled clinical trial. Pain 2008;136:271–80.

Index

Page numbers followed by b refer to boxes, f to figures, and t to tables.

Treatment credibility and engagement, 101–105, 176–177
  biomedical orientation of patients, 101–102
  case conceptualization and rationale, 103
  didactic teaching supporting, 104–105
  goal setting and life values, 177
  graded exposure for CRPS-I, 149–150
  graded exposure vs. graded activity efficacy, 137–138
  medical examination establishing, 103
  psycho-educational format and, 177
  treatment dropouts and, 102, 106, 162, 164, 176
  treatment preferences for musculoskeletal pain, 176
  understanding of fear-avoidance model, 104
Treatment goals, determining, 80–81, 82b
TSK. *See* Tampa Scale for Kinesiophobia (TSK)

U

Unconditioned responses, 27–33
  physiological arousal, 28–29
  in respondent conditioning, 33
  types of, 26
Unconditioned stimulus (US), 26, 33

V

Validation, in exposure therapy, 180
Validity of studies, 115
Verbal instruction
  as exposure delivery method, 178
  pain-related fear and, 36–37, 55–56
Virtual reality, exposure using, 91
Visual analogue scale (VAS), 131, 164
Visual analysis of data, 121–122

W

Walking Stairs Questionnaire (WSQ), 149
Whiplash injury, 152–155, 153f, 154f
Withdrawal from stimulus, 26, 173
Written information, value of, 76–77

Johan W.S. Vlaeyen, PhD, is a professor in the Research Group Health Psychology, Faculty of Psychology and Educational Sciences, University of Leuven, Belgium, and at the Department of Clinical Psychological Science, Faculty of Psychology and Neuroscience, Maastricht University, The Netherlands. He received an honorary doctorate from Örebro University, Sweden. His research interests include the affective and motivational mechanisms of task interference due to persistent pain. Vlaeyen and his team developed exposure-based therapy for patients with chronic pain. They have conducted randomized controlled trials as well as replicated single-case experiments to evaluate the effects of behavioral interventions in chronic pain.

Stephen J. Morley, MPhil, PhD, is a professor of clinical psychology and director of the clinical psychology training program at the Institute of Health Sciences, University of Leeds, United Kingdom. He is also a practicing clinical psychologist at St James' University Hospital, Leeds. His research interests include the effects of pain on self-identity and the development of clinical methods for evaluating the effectiveness of psychological treatments for chronic pain. He is section editor of the European Journal of Pain

Steven J. Linton, PhD, is professor of clinical psychology at the School of Law, Psychology, and Social Work and research director of the Center for Health and Medical Psychology (CHAMP) at Örebrö University, Örebrö, Sweden. His research interests include the role of psychological factors in sleep disorders, ways to match psychological interventions to the specific needs of patients with chronic pain, and behavioral therapies for restoring function and quality of life in patients with disability from persistent musculoskeletal pain.

Katja Boersma, PhD, is associate professor at the School of Law, Psychology, and Social Work and a researcher at the Center for Health and Medical Psychology, Örebrö University, Örebrö, Sweden. Her research interests include biopsychosocial aspects of pain, including fear-avoidance and catastrophizing.

Jeroen de Jong, PhD, is a movement scientist, behavior therapist, and researcher at the Department of Rehabilitation, Maastricht University Hospital, Maastricht, The Netherlands. Along with Vlaeyen, de Jong is recognized as one of the founders of graded exposure in vivo therapy in chronic pain.